Faith, Love, and Laughter
Surviving Cancer

Candace D. Eide

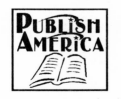

PublishAmerica
Baltimore

ISBN: 1-4241-9888-7
PUBLISHED BY PUBLISHAMERICA, LLLP
www.publishamerica.com
Baltimore

Printed in the United States of America

Thank you Leon, Chris, Kelly, Rita, Larry, Ron, Judy, Billie, Susan and Midge for being there with me for the worst of times and the best of times.

Chapter One
Meet the Eides

This was very infiltrated carcinomas with the entire auxiliary fat pad infiltrated with tumor, and pathology report showed infiltrating duct carcinoma, poorly differentiated and tumor and carcinoma metastasis to fifteen of fifteen ancillary lymph nodes with massive tumor involvement of all lymph node levels.
Prognosis at this point is guarded as this is a Stage II+ situation.

* * * * * * * * * *

There are so many times as we go through life we are hit with a challenge. Some are easy to get through, and some test us to the brink of despair. As we face each challenge, we deal with it as best as we can with the information we have at the moment and then we forget about it. Not totally, of course. We store it in the very recesses of our mind just in case we have to deal with that particular challenge again and then we have an idea of what worked and what didn't work in the past. Generally as a rule we don't dwell on it unless it rears its ugly head again. But of course there is always an exception to every rule. There is that one challenge that hits you square and takes your breath away. You don't see it coming. You are never prepared for it. And no matter how much time passes you never forget it.

My name is Candace Eide (pronounced i-dee). I am a cancer survivor. This is my story. It is about surviving cancer. It is about the discoveries, the frustration, the fears, the pain, the regrets and most of all the joys I experienced.

I am married to Leon, and we have two children: a son Chris, a daughter Kelly, and a cat named Katie. When Leon and I met it was love at first sight. I was seventeen, in high school, and he was nineteen, attending the local community college. We married young. We are among the lucky ones. It has been and is a great relationship, despite my grandmother's warning that mixed marriages are difficult. He is Catholic and I am Lutheran! I still get a chuckle out of that.

However, for as well as we get along our personalities are very different. I live in the moment and tend to get excited about little things, and he is reserved, quiet and shy. *Someone told me once that if you tied my hands behind my back I wouldn't be able to talk!* I get bored easily and enjoy creating a wee bit of chaos every once in a while just to keep things interesting! He likes things to run smoothly without any trouble. I love to dance. He prefers listening to music. And I am an eternal optimist. I always look for the positive in every situation. Leon just takes things as they come.

Like I said, we are quite different, but we compliment each other nicely. Both of us have strong family values, love our children and family, adore our friends, and enjoy outdoor activities. And we both have the same weakness: we both like to gamble. We have talked about going to Las Vegas for years, but we never think we can afford it. It's the value thing…pay bills, buy food and clothing, meet the children's needs, and if there is any money left over, go out to dinner every once in a while.

At the time of this story Chris was eighteen. He had graduated from high school in the fall of 1989 and was attending the local community college. Kelly was sixteen and a sophomore in high school. She played basketball and volleyball. Both children were living at home. It seemed on a daily basis Kelly was urging Chris to get an apartment so she could have his bedroom!

Leon's mother, three brothers, and sister lived in Missoula, Montana. His dad had passed away some years ago. I have one brother. He and his family lived in North Dakota.

My mother and father were divorced. It wasn't a pleasant experience. Divorce for my parents' generation was uncommon.

There was a big stigma attached to you if you were divorced. My mother worried about that a lot. But as with many a challenge, this too passed. My dad moved to North Dakota, and my mother remained in Glendive. It was a good thing that there was a lot of distance between them.

My story takes place in Glendive, a rural community in eastern Montana. Glendive is a friendly community with about 5000 people in the city and about the same in the surrounding area. The economic base is dependent on farming. The Yellowstone River divides the city. Clay hills and prairie plains surround it. There is a state park called Makoshika, and it is famous for dinosaur excavation. Glendive is located approximately forty miles from the North Dakota border. It is at the very eastern edge of the third largest state in the nation. The largest populated city in Montana is Billings (approximately 90,000 people) and it is about 220 miles away. The good news is Glendive is located along the interstate highway, so it's relatively easy to get to where you want to go.

Glendive is a good place to raise children. It has some of the finest schools in the state, including a small community college. There is a clinic and a hospital. Both facilities are good but not without their challenges. For example, it is a struggle for rural communities to find doctors and get them to stay for any length of time. Most of them come from urban areas. They initially move to acquire experience and then leave after a year or two, or they find their families simply cannot adjust to living in a rural community. If they do manage to stay they soon find themselves overbooked, overworked, and burned out in a short period of time.

The upside to living in a small community reminds me of the theme song on the TV show, *Cheers*, "*Where everybody knows your name.*" Sooner or later you have probably spoken to everyone who lives there—if not at some basketball, volleyball, or baseball game, surely at a children's program.

Here are some sayings about small-town life: "You know you live in a small town when you cannot walk for exercise because every car that passes you stops to see if you need a ride." "You dial a wrong number and talk for twenty minutes, and then the person gives you the right number." And last but not least, "You know you live in a small town when you miss church on Sunday and receive a get-well card the next day."

The best part of living in a small town is friendships run deep. I read something once or maybe someone told me that you are blessed if you have one true friend in your lifetime. I have been blessed. I have three wonderful friends. They are Billie, Midge, and Susan. We have been friends since the seventh grade and are often referred to as "the girls." Everyone knows who we are. Our friendship has survived our teenage years, weddings, pregnancies, divorces, and a whole lot of what-were-you-thinking? stuff." Over the years distance has separated us by someone either moving away or getting sidetracked by raising a family. But we have always somehow, someway, managed to reconnect. Our friendship is steadfast and has lasted through the test of time. We remain the best of friends today. There is a saying, "A friend is someone who knows you but loves you anyway." The reality is, we must remain friends. We have no choice. We have much too much personal knowledge about each other! Some might call it blackmail material, but I prefer to think of it as general information that we have stored for future reference!

Leon and I have also acquired "married friends" independent from "the girls." They are Rita and Larry. I met Rita at work. We discovered we lived in the same neighborhood, so we started a carpool. Through Rita and Larry we were introduced to Ron and Judy. Rita, Larry, and Judy had attended the same high school where Ron had taught English. Larry and Rita were Ron's students. At the time I met Rita I was looking for a babysitter. Rita heard Judy was starting a daycare, and it just so happened that they, too, lived just down the street and around the corner. It was perfect. We have become such good friends. When the six of us get together—watch out! We are quite a six-pack, and the time we have spent together is, well, priceless!

Another advantage to living in a small town is that whenever there is crisis, "like a good neighbor" the community comes together.

Everyone pitches in to help fix whatever is broken. Generosity runs abundant.

The biggest disadvantage to living in a small town is…people know waaaay too much! You sneeze, and people at work the next day will bless you, ask you how your allergies are, or say they heard were you were catching a cold! There are no secrets. In other words, if you don't know what you are doing somebody else does! It all gets around sooner or later.

Leon and I are typical working class. We live from paycheck to paycheck with nothing to spare at the end of the week. Most of my working career has been in the non-profit sector, which by the name itself indicates it is not a high-paying field. But my work experience has been wonderful. I have learned a lot of basic principles that have carried me through some interesting challenges, including cancer. You see, I have a belief system that attitude, being grateful, and how you treat yourself are keys to living a happy and fulfilling life.

For example, two words that I have tried to eliminate from my vocabulary or at least use very, very sparingly are "problem" and "stupid." The connotations of those two words can leave you feeling helpless or worthless. Let's face it; life in general can be tough enough, but when you use words that leave you with a feeling of worthlessness, surviving just gets harder.

In 1990 I added two words to my vocabulary that I have used regularly…"cancer survivor." I spent one full year—365 days—in survival mode. This is my version, my truth if you will, on living with cancer.

⋆⇀⇒⇐↼⋆

Your living is determined not so much by what life brings to you as by the attitude you bring to life; not so much by what happens to you as by the way your mind looks at what happens.

—John Homer Miller

Chapter Two
Looky, Looky, What I Found!

My story begins on a typical frigid winter night in February. The forecast called for an arctic front to move in, and it did. The temperature hung in at ten degrees below zero with a wind-chill factor of thirty-two degrees below zero. "Did you know that skin can freeze in less than ten minutes when exposed to this kind of cold?" Leon and I had returned from a quick trip to the grocery store. It was a short trip, and consequently the car never had a chance to warm up. I was chilled to the bone, and I hate being cold! For me there is nothing worse than that bitter, icy-cold feeling that seeps deep into your very being. Everything seems to ache.

I decided a hot soaker was just what I needed to warm me up. It was great. The steam was rising as I lay in the tub enjoying the heat that was permeating through my bones. But unfortunately after an hour or so of letting the warm water drain and refilling it with hot water, I had finally used up all the hot water. And, as usual, all good things must come to an end—the water in the tub was getting cold also.

I decided before getting out of the tub to do a self breast-examination. It wasn't something that I did very often. After all, I was only thrity-seven years old, and breast cancer or any kind of cancer rarely crossed my mind. Plus I was on a roll. I was healthy except for an occasional cold. I was feeling really good, and things were going great. I was too busy working and raising a family to be interrupted with such a thing. After all, I had two children and a husband and cat who needed me. And as far as I was concerned cancer was something you dealt with when you were much older, like fifty-something. To be perfectly honest, if I did think about the big "C" I was more concerned about getting lung cancer. I hate to admit it, but I was a smoker. Over the last five years or so, there had been more and more information coming out about the awful side-effects of smoking. I had tried to quit numerous times—you know, the New Year's resolution thing—but never could get it done! The fact was I never worried much about that either. Both my parents were heavy smokers, and they were both alive, doing well, and over fifty! My reality—my belief was you got cancer when you were older. Chicken pox, tonsillitis, etc., were things you got when you were younger, arthritis and cancer were things you got when you were much older. You know, fifty-something!

Being right handed I started out with my left side. I raised my arm and began with a circular motion, starting at the top of the breast and working clockwise, and then gently pressing on the nipple area. Since I don't have fibrous breasts there were no unusual bumps or lumps. I moved to my right side. Again I started at the top and worked my way around and then to the nipple. I paused. "Hmmm." I repeated the procedure again. And there it was—again. *Yes, there definitely is something under the nipple I have never noticed before.* I calmly got out of the tub, although I have to admit my heart was racing a little. I dried myself off and put my pajamas on. *I wonder how Leon is going to react to this?*

Leon was downstairs watching TV, and the kids were in their bedrooms getting ready for bed. I went downstairs and sat on the couch next to him. I looked at him and said, "I need your undivided attention." He looked at me. He knew when I needed his undivided attention something was up.

"I think I have a problem." I said calmly. "I was taking a bath and decided to do a self-breast examination, and I found something under my right nipple."

He continued to look at me and said, "You make a doctor's appointment first thing in the morning. Don't be messing around and put it off." I don't like going to the doctor and have a tendency to wait it out as long as I can.

"Hon, I want you to check to see if you feel anything." I said. And he did.

He tried to hide the surprise in his eyes as he felt "it." "Candace, you make a doctor's appointment first thing in the morning," he repeated. "You cannot put this off. I want you to get this checked."

"What if it's cancerous?" I asked, still feeling fairly calm. "What if I lose a breast?"

"Candace, I didn't marry you for your boobs. Whether you have two breasts, one breast, or none, it won't make any difference. I will still love you as much as I love you now."

I am not sure what reaction I was expecting from him. Leon and I have always had a good relationship. Over the years, we had survived a few challenges still intact and loving each other, but I had a strong feeling this was going to be completely different. I needed to know he was going to be there. I needed to be assured that if I lost a part of me, no matter what part it may be, it would not make a difference in his feelings for me.

For the record I am not beautiful by any means. Okay as far as looks go. Men don't go "googily-eyed" when I walk by, but they don't get sick to their stomachs either. And as far as my body goes—when I was younger…much, much younger, I had a decent shape. In fact I was nominated "Miss Legs" my senior year in high school. But after two children, becoming a healthy connoisseur of foods, and hitting the "thirty" mark, the best way to describe my body now is—a stick, a beanpole, a straight line—in other words, the curves are simply gone!

Also at this point in my life I have gained enough confidence in myself to know that I am more than a body. My body is a small part of who I really am. I am a person. I am a good person who loves unselfishly and cares deeply about the people around me. For me personally, if losing a breast is the option for living, you can have it—take it. As far as I am concerned it has no value.

At least that is how I felt at this very moment. Circumstances have a funny way of changing your belief systems!

There wasn't much more to be said. We spent the rest of the evening staring at the TV not really paying attention to what was on. We were both absorbed in our own thoughts. We finally said good night to the kids and made our way upstairs to go to bed.

The bed was freezing. We snuggled together, Leon gently holding me in his arms. "Good night. Love you," he said. "Love you," I answered back. Every night before we go to sleep we say, "Love you," even when we are upset with each other. It's a habit we had gotten into doing since the first day we were married.

After a while I could tell by his breathing that he had finally fallen asleep. I closed my eyes, but the realization that I had found something kept my mind from shutting down. I couldn't shake the impending feeling of doom. It was a long and restless night.

* * * * * * * * * * * *

The alarm broke the silence and Leon reached to turn it off. I was glad it was time to get up. I hadn't slept well, if at all. All kinds of stuff kept running through my mind, you know: the "What if this?" and the "What if that?" stuff that keeps your mind from shutting down.

The best way for me to describe the "What if this" and "What if that's" is—they are little demons. They sneak into your subconscious mind and lie in wait until you are alone and afraid about one thing or another. And then, like ghostly whispers of smoke, they invade your thoughts. They play cruel mind games by creating imaginary worst-case scenarios that cause unnecessary anxiety and worry. They paralyze you in fear to what may happen. And those are the key words—you think or picture in your mind things that may happen when you are fearful or feeling stress. And they are very, very creative. The "what if's" feed on pain, panic, and fear. They are dangerous, and like a cancer, if left unchecked, will grow and consume you, causing you endless and unwarranted stress to your physical and mental well-being.

It is Monday, February fifth, and true to the weather forecast, cold: plain and simple. The furnace was working overtime trying to keep the temperature in the house a toasty sixty-eight degrees. I tried to be my cheerful self. I made breakfast as usual, talked about trivial things, and sent the children out the door to their destinations. Leon again, before he went out the door to work, gently insisted that I make a doctor's appointment.

I headed for work. It was very cold outside. I hate being cold. But I didn't notice it as much as I had the night before. I was distracted with other things on my mind. The demons were hard at work.

Once at work, I busied myself with little to-do things until I knew the doctor's office was open. I had one challenge, though. I didn't have a doctor. My doctor had retired, and I hadn't needed one since his retirement. There were two long-standing doctors still practicing, but they were getting up in retirement age also. Plus their caseloads were full, and they didn't want to take any new patients. I thumbed through the hospital directory and stopped on Dr. Shorn's name. He was new to the area, and as far as the rumor mill went, I hadn't heard anything bad about him. So I figured I would take a chance and hope there would be a good doctor-patient relationship. I figured he was as good as any, and I'd give him a chance.

I called to request an appointment. The receptionist asked in what regards I wanted to see the doctor?

I said, matter of factly, "I had found a lump and wanted it checked."

She asked me when I could come in. "Whenever I can." I said. I had an appointment for that afternoon.

I had barely hung up the phone when it rang. "Candace, you have a telephone call on line two," the receptionist announced on the intercom.

"Hi, this is Candace," I said in my most professional voice.

"Did you make a doctor's appointment?" a man's voice asked demandingly.

"No 'Hi, how are ya, whatcha doing?'" I asked.

"No. A simple question that requires a simple answer," my husband replied impatiently. "Did you make a doctor's appointment?"

"You are always to the point—never any small talk." I replied. "Yes, I made an appointment for this afternoon."

"Do you want me to go with you?" he asked.

"No, that's okay. They probably won't do too much anyway. Most likely I will have to come back and do some tests. Anyhow, you know me. 'I am woman, hear me roar!' 'I can bring home the bacon, fry it up in a pan, and never let you forget you're the man!'" I joked.

"Yeah, yeah I know. I've heard it all before. Call me when you know something, okay?" he said firmly.

"You'll be the first—no, the doctor will be the first, so you will be the second; no, I will be the second. You could be the third person depending on if the nurse finds out before I tell you," I said, trying to lighten the mood.

"Candace," he interrupted

"Yes," I said back.

"Call me when you know something, please!"

"I promise." There was a short pause.

"I love you," he said quietly.

"I love you too."

I hung up the phone and just sat there. *Like a puff of smoke wafting through the air, the demons began their ascent into my thoughts.* I shook them off and pulled some work out. I tried hard to stay focused, but my thoughts kept wandering off. *Damn those demons!*

"I must concentrate," I said to myself as I reread what I had just written over again for the fifth time. I could tell it was going to be a long, long morning.

* * * * * * * * * * * *

I arrived at the clinic early. It's a habit I have gotten into. I am always early to wherever I am going and most often the first one to arrive. Today it was a good thing. I was a new patient. When I checked in with the receptionist she handed me a clipboard with a form to fill out. There were questions front and back. It was a long form.

Let's see, first question, list any childhood diseases? I wrote I had a ruptured appendix when I was five, the German measles at seven.

Then I remembered when I was eleven years old. That was an interesting year! It started with the chicken pox and then mumps, first on my right side and then on the left side; couldn't have it all at once, of course; and ended with an acute glomerulonephritis, commonly referred to as Bright's disease. It affects the kidneys. In fact my right kidney stopped working for a while, and I spent three months in a hospital in bed. But that wasn't the worst part. The worst part was I could not have chocolate! Seriously. Think about it. I'm eleven years old, a girl, and could not have chocolate! What were they thinking? And since I was sick most of my eleventh year I missed a lot of school and had to repeat fifth grade. After that dreadful year there wasn't anything unusual to report except an occasional cold or touch of flu although I know the chocolate thing scarred me forever!

List any illnesses as an adult. The question becomes…are you considered an adult at eighteen? *I was married and had a baby, so yes I was an adult at eighteen.* A few months after my first child was born, I developed hepatitis and spent a week in the hospital in isolation. I have my own theories on how I ended up with hepatitis, but that is another story. The interesting part of this story was all my family and friends who I had had prior contact with in the previous week or so had to have a shot. My immediate family, "the girls," and their families all had to get vaccinated! They were not happy-campers! I have also discovered that none of them have long-term memory loss because they still bring it up today!

List any pregnancies. I wrote down I had two pregnancies and two miscarriages. Both pregnancies went fine. Both miscarriages were devastating, especially the first one. I had started bleeding in my third month. The doctor wanted to try bed rest for a few days before doing a DNC. On the third day of my hospital stay Leon was sitting with me in my room. He was dozing off and on. I watched him slip in and out of sleep trying to stay awake, thinking to myself how cute he was. Then I felt myself slowly drifting away…far, far away. I was going to a place that was warm and different in a way that's hard to describe. I was gently floating toward this glowing aura of light. It was such a warm feeling, like a soft and gentle caress touching my body. It was beautiful and mesmerizing! I slowly kept drawing closer and closer to it.

Then suddenly, I felt this slap across my face. "Candace, Candace! Wake up! Can you hear me?"

Go away, I am almost there! I begged silently. *I can almost touch it!*

Again, a slap across the face, and none too gentle, I might add. "Candace, Candace! Wake up! Can you hear me?" I heard again.

Noooo! I thought as I moved away from the light.

And then I heard my mother's voice. "Candace, Candace! Wake up! Can you hear me?" she pleaded.

The light vanished, and I opened my eyes. My mother, Leon, and the nurse, who had the nerve to slap me in the face numerous times, were standing over me.

"When did you get here, Mom?" I asked nonchalantly, as if I had just awakened from a nap.

"Just now," she said. "And I think just in the nick of time."

As my mother tells it, when she came into my room she found Leon asleep in the chair. She looked at me and got a little concerned because she didn't think I looked quite right. I was too pale, and my breathing seemed very shallow. So she pulled the emergency alarm in the bathroom and then went out in the hall and yelled, "Something is wrong!" This outburst caused my husband to wake up suddenly. He was slightly disoriented when the nurse came running in. The nurse looked the situation over, took my pulse, decided Mom was right and started slapping me on the cheeks. I was rudely awakened!

I have read about people who have seen the "white light." My belief about this experience was for a brief moment God was considering calling me home. Why, at that moment, I don't know. For whatever reason He decided to let me stay a while longer. Some day, not too soon I hope, I will ask Him what changed His mind.

Ah…back to the form. Any known allergies? No. Any known family members with cancer? Yes, my grandmother on my father's side, two uncles and two aunts on my mother's side. If yes, list: I wrote breast cancer, lung cancer, ovarian cancer, and lymphoma…just to name a few.

CANDACE D. EIDE

I looked at what I had just written and realized that the numbers were stacked against me. More importantly, everyone I knew in my family who had cancer, had died from it. Yes, they were older but nonetheless, they had died from cancer.

"Candace." I heard the nurse call my name. I looked up and there was a familiar face. It was the same nurse who had worked in the clinic with my doctor who had retired. I looked at her for a moment. I must have had that deer-in-the-headlight look, because I was debating if I should run as fast as I could and get the hell out of there or stay for the verdict. I had a strong premonition this wasn't going to turn out very good. And since I am a betting person I didn't like the odds—at all.

"Candace," she repeated. "Come with me." Slowly I stood up and handed her the clipboard with the form that I had completed. "It's nice to see you again. It has been awhile. How are you today?" she smiled at me.

Are you crazy? Can't you see that I am scared out of my wits? I wanted to scream but instead I said, "I'm fine." Smiling back at her.

We stopped by the scale to weight me. She moved the little weights back and forth until they balanced on 145 pounds. I grunted. Hmmmm…I had gained thirty-three pounds with my second child and had topped off at 153 pounds. Since I have hit the "thirty" mark, it seemed that each year I had put on a couple of extra unwanted pounds. *I must do something about this weight gain before it really gets out of hand.* I thought.

"Follow me," she said as she pointed to examining room number three. She took my temperature and blood pressure and requested that I remove all my clothes except my underwear and socks and change into what they commonly refer as a gown *it's certainly not what I visualize when I hear the word gown!* "The doctor will be in shortly," she said as she left the room.

Now I gotta tell ya I am not dumb by any means but it took me about five minutes to figure out how to put that silly gown together! I don't know how many times I had to unsnap it one way and snap it together another way before I finally got it right! My next dilemma was—am

I supposed to put the opening to the back or to the front? She didn't say. I'm here to have my breasts examined *and while I am here, why not my head?* so logically I would think he would want it to the front. But if I remember correctly I've never put the opening to the front. I have always put it to the back so maybe that's what I should do. But when he examines me, he will have to lift up the entire gown. I hate this already and I really, really hate this gown!

The good news was that I had been so distracted by the gown that I had completely forgotten the real reason why I was there! Finally after making an executive decision, I put the opening to the back, grabbed a magazine, sat down, totally exhausted, and waited for the doctor.

The only sound in the room was the ticking of the second hand on the clock. Tick, tick, tick...minutes seemed like hours, hours seemed like days, after I thumbed through my fourth, fifth, no sixth magazine! *I thought she said the doctor would be here shortly?* The wait in the examining room always seems excruciatingly long.

I hate waiting especially in doctor's offices. I figured by the time the doctor did get in to see you, you were already feeling better just because so much time has passed waiting. I have to admit that over the years I had a tendency to wait out whatever "illness or thing" I had as long as I could before seeing a doctor. And most of the time it worked. I figured it saved me lots of money on doctor's visits and prescriptions I wouldn't take. I guess that was why Leon was insistent on me making a doctor's appointment and keeping it this time.

Dang, now I remember why I am here. For a brief moment the gown fiasco had me sidetracked, but reality was back. Finally Dr. Shorn entered and extended his hand, "Hi," he said. "I'm Dr. Shorn. Candace, right?"

"Yes," I said offering my hand. I hoped it wasn't sweaty. My palms get sweaty when I am nervous. I looked at him and he smiled. He had a nice smile.

For me, finding a good doctor is very personal. After all, you trust this person with...well the whole you. This person will most likely have more intimate knowledge about you than anyone else. I believe it is human nature to try to hide your imperfections from others, yes even our spouse. It is the doctor that sees you when you are most vulnerable and knows your imperfections. You must trust that person to fix you up and make you feel better. But what I hate the most is that feeling of weakness when I am sick. I hate that fwhen you have to depend on someone to help make it better. But today was different. I have to admit I had the feeling I was in the right place. I relaxed.

"According to your chart, you are concerned about something you found while doing a breast examination. I'll have you get up on the table." I grasped the back of the gown and proceeded to the examining table. "Lie down and raise your hand above your head," he said as he unsnapped the sleeve on the left side of the gown. *"Ah, now I understand the snaps!"*

I averted my eyes and tried to find something else to look at while he began his examination. I happened to look up and on the ceiling there was a poster on the four food groups. I tried to focus on it as he performed the same circular motions I had done the night before. He gently pulled my left arm down and snapped the sleeve back in place. He moved to the right side. Again he said, "Raise your arm above your head," as he unsnapped the right sleeve. He preformed the circular motions, gently pressing and then he stopped. I wonder if he could hear or feel my heart beating because it was thumping pretty good! He repeated the procedure again. He asked me to sit up. "Well," he said, "there is something definitely there. I think we need a picture. I will set up a mammogram for you. Have you ever had a mammogram before?"

"No." I said. *Listen I am only thirty-seven years old, and the articles I read and the news reports on TV said I didn't need to get a baseline mammogram until I was forty. I am supposed to have at least three more years before I have to have a mammogram. It's not right! I was misinformed by the information. I believed what was reported. It's not fair. I was lied to!*

"I was under the impression that the recommended age for a baseline mammogram was age forty?" I asked, slightly perturbed.

"Yes and no. It's different for each woman. It depends on your health, your family history, and your insurance company." He replied smiling. "You can get dressed, and I'll have Betty set up an appointment for you," he said as he left the room. I sat there calmly watching him close the door, leaving me alone. I got up from the exam table and began getting dressed. I remembered years ago a colleague of mine had gone to the doctor for a suspicious lump that had been determined cancerous. I remember her telling me the worst part was the doctor told her it was cancer and then left the room. There she sat all alone, had just been told she had cancer, didn't know if she was going to live or die and the doctor immediately left the room. She said it was awful. She wasn't sure if she should scream, cry or get mad. All she knew was that she was more frightened than she had been in her entire life. She figured he was uncomfortable because she was a nurse and a colleague. Regardless she felt she deserved more than his back leaving the room.

The door opened and Dr. Shorn entered interrupting my thoughts. He sat down at the little desk in the corner of the room. "You have an appointment for a mammogram at 10:00 a.m. on Friday the ninth," he said. "I also made an appointment for you to see me at 2:00 p.m. Do you have any questions?"

"Ummm, I don't know." I was caught off guard. "I guess the million-dollar question is...do I have cancer?" I heard myself say out loud.

"I don't know. I'll have a better idea after the mammogram. There is definitely a mass under your right nipple, but if it is cancer, I cannot confirm it at this time. Once I get the results back from the films, I'll be able to give you more information. I know this may sound trivial, but try not to worry too much about it. Go through your normal routine, okay? It could be nothing. Do you have any other questions?"

"I don't think so, at least not at this time," I answered.

"Okay, I will see you back on Friday afternoon." As a gesture of reassurance, he gently patted my shoulder as he walked out the room. I sat there for a moment. *Well, off to my normal routine as if there is nothing wrong.*

I left his office surprisingly calm. With a half-hearted attempt I convinced myself that I was not going to worry about it! *You can kiss my putootie, demons! I have no time for you now.* I took a deep breath and then it hit me…the cold air as it infiltrated my lungs and stung my eyes as I opened the front door and a strong feeling that it was going to be much easier said than done.

I went back to work and called Leon with what news I had. There really wasn't much to report. I dug out some work but had difficulty concentrating on it. I hid my anxiety. I did not want my co-workers to get suspicious. I was not ready to share my fears with anyone quite yet. I busied myself doing nothing. Intuition told me I was going have a lot of distractions in the in the coming weeks.

* * * * * * * * * * * * *

I believe in God with my whole heart and I talk to God every day. Sometimes I talk to Him frequently depending on what is going on! I wish I could say I could quote you scripture upon scripture but I can't. I just know I believe in Him and the power of prayer. It is comforting to know that He is with me always. I cannot imagine living life without the grace of God!

Every night before I go to sleep I tell Leon and my children I love them and then I pray. First I say the Lord's Prayer. Then I pray for the forgiveness of the sins I have committed that day. I pray that He watches over and forgives my children of their sins. I pray that He touches their hearts and souls and guides them so that they make smart choices. I pray for forgiveness of my family and friends. Then I pray for the sin in the world that at times can seem so overwhelming. Last but not least, I thank God for all wonderful blessings that I have in my life. Everyday I make a point to be grateful for something. Sometimes it is a major gratefulness and sometimes it is as simple as the warmth of Leon's hand holding mine.

My prayers this week included Dr. Shorn. *Thank you, God, for helping me choose Dr. Shorn.* I was grateful that I was guided to Dr. Shorn. He made me feel comfortable and had a genuine caring nature about him. Most importantly, I felt that I could trust him with my life. This was a major gratefulness, because I contend that I am here today partly because of Dr. Shorn and the choices he made regarding my diagnosis.

⊷⟟⟢⊷

Oh what a cause of thankfulness it is that we have a gracious God to go to on all occasions! Use and enjoy this privilege and you can never be miserable. Oh, what an unspeakable privilege is prayer!

—Lady Maxwell

Chapter Three
A Picture Is Worth Many, Many Lumps

I am amazed at how quickly things can go from honky-dory, to a complete disaster in a blink of an eye. It is that moment in your life when change hits you square and takes your breath away. Things are never the same again. In one brief moment, less than a minute—your life can be turned upside down, literally. What you knew to be true in one minute, can be so different in the next and it all happens in less than a minute. WOW.

It was Friday the 9th and I was calmly sitting in the hospital waiting room awaiting my turn for a mammogram. In the short time I had arrived I had spoke with three acquaintances regarding why we were there. One woman hadn't been feeling well and the doctor wanted some blood work done. But she assured us they didn't think it was serious. One had stepped off the curb and twisted his ankle. He was in for x-rays to see if there was a hair-line fracture. Another was waiting to have her annual mammogram.

That was a good one, I thought as I was frantically trying to come up with a good excuse. I told a fib and said I was in for an annual physical too.

After all I wanted to be the first to know if I had the "big C." I didn't want it floating around town, "Did you hear? Poor Candace has cancer." I wanted to be the one to tell everyone. It was my disease and I should get first dibs at spreading the news.

The waiting room is located in the lower level of the hospital. There is a common area where you wait to have blood work done, x-rays and respiratory therapy. Each department is located in a different hallway.

The nurse or technician from each particular department enters the common area and calls your name.

I watched as Karen, the x-ray technician (an acquaintance from high school) walked down the hall. *Please call me,* I thought. *I have had about all chit-chat I can take today.* I am now in the need-to-get-this-over-as-soon-as-possible phase of this process. It had been four days since my visit with Dr. Shorn and I am tired of my so-called normal routine. I haven't slept well and little things were starting to get to me besides not knowing was getting old.

"Hi, Candace," she said as she motioned for me. "How are you today?" she asked as I walked towards her.

"This is my first mammogram, so a little nervous, I think!" I answered back. "From what I've heard and seen, this is not going to be much fun."

She laughed. "The good news is it only takes a couple of minutes or so. Of course it will seem like the longest minutes ever! You will be fine, I'm sure." She pointed to the room. "You need to take everything off from your waist up, and then put this gown on. Also if you have deodorant on please wipe it off with this cloth, and then you can throw it away. While you are waiting, here is some information for you to read. I will be back in a minute," she said as she handed me the gown and reading material. And then she left the room.

Uck...please, not the gown again! I looked at it. *It's time I take control of this situation. If I can't handle a silly little gown I am in big trouble.* Snap, snap, and in less than thirty seconds I had my clothes off, and the gown was on! I was so proud. I wiped the deodorant off with the cloth and threw it away. *I wonder why you can't wear deodorant,* I thought to myself.

I looked at the brochure on how to prepare for a mammogram that Karen had laid on the desk.

Do not wear deodorant, talcum powder or lotion under your arms or on your breasts on the day of the exam. These can appear on the mammogram as calcium spots.

Well, now I know!

Describe any breast symptoms or problems to the technologist performing the exam.

Does she know why I am here? Did Dr. Shorn inform her or should I tell her? I wonder what would happen if she puts too much pressure down on "that thing"? Will it burst and spread? I better tell her just to be on the safe side.

Ask when your results will be available; do not assume the results are normal if you do not hear from your doctor or the mammography facility.

I have an appointment this afternoon, so I assume...but no, I shouldn't assume, that Dr Shorn will have the results by then, right? I was getting confused.

Karen entered the room. "Okay, are you ready?" she asked as she guided me to the mammography machine.

"Take your left arm out of the gown," she said.

"Karen, I don't know if you know the reason I am here. I had found a lump, and Dr. Shorn wants me to have it checked."

"Yes," she said, "there was a note on your file."

"I have a silly question. Can it break and spread if you put too much pressure on it?"

"No, in fact I will want to compress it as far as I can so we can get a good picture." She reached for my left breast. "My hands might be a little cold," she said. *Might—be a little cold! Oh...my...gawd, her hands were freezing!* She grabbed my left breast, pulling and stretching it, as she placed it on the platform. I tried not to flinch, *but oh...my...gawd her hands were ice cold!*

"Sorry about the cold hands," she said again, as she concentrated on getting my breast positioned. "And the platform might be cold too! I have been meaning to get a heating pad or something to warm it up, but I keep forgetting."

Well, this is just plain ridiculous! I cringed as she laid my pulled and stretched boob on the icy platform, and then said, "Now reach up and grab onto the side of the machine and hold it. Now relax a little."

Okay, I give her credit. She has a great sense of humor

"Now I am going to add a little pressure…hold it…hold it…tell me when it gets uncomfortable." *Ah, too late. That happened when I walked into the room!*

"Hold it; okay, hold your breath and," she said as she exited behind a glass shield to take the picture.

Let's see, according to the information I read, the technical version of how a mammogram procedure is performed goes something like this. During a mammogram a technologist will position your breast in the mammography unit.

Note, there is no mention of icy cold hands or machine.

Your breast will be placed on a special platform and compressed with a paddle.

A paddle? Let's call it what it really is…a vice, plain and simple.

The technologist will gradually compress your breast.

In other words prolong the agony as long as possible.

You will feel pressure on your breast as it is squeezed by the compressor.

Squeezed is the operative word here. Picture a balloon, and you want to pop it. You squeeze it, and you feel the resistance, but you keep squeezing it and squeezing it, applying more and more pressure, and suddenly—POP!

You may experience some discomfort.

Are you serious? "Some discomfort?" I am quite sure that is not an adequate description of your breast being flattened like a pancake.

"Now let's do the right side," she said.

The good news was her hands were much warmer, and the heat from my left breast had warmed the platform up as well. Could things get any better?

"I'll have you wait until I check the films to be sure the picture is good. Then you can get dressed," she said as she left the room. I quickly double checked my breasts to make sure they reverted back to their natural form. Whew, there didn't seem to be any permanent damage. I calmly waited, trying to concentrate on something else by rereading the material she had given me. The challenge was I had trouble retaining the information I was reading. *The demons kept reappearing and distracting* me. I tried to clear my mind. *I hope this doesn't take long,* I said to myself.

The door opened but it was not Karen. It was Dr. Benjamen. He was the radiologist. I recognized him from his picture in the paper. He was originally from India and talk around town was he was one of the best in his field. Glendive was lucky to have him.

"I looked at your films, and I want to do an ultrasound."

At least I think that is what he said! Although he spoke English he had a thick Indian accent and spoke very rapidly.

"It will give us a better picture." He motioned me to follow him. I obediently stood up and followed him to another room. "Lie down here," he said as he pointed to the bed. I did what he asked.

In translation he said something to the effect of, "I'm going to apply some conducting gel on this area. It helps with the transmission of the sound waves." He explained, "It will be a little cold and wet." I clearly understood what he meant as I flinched when he dabbed the cold gel around my breast!

Sheez...can't they warm this stuff up? I really hate cold. When I am done here I'm going to find a suggestion box or maybe talk with the administrator or someone and tell them to start warming things up around here! This is ridiculous.

He turned on the ultrasound machine. "Ultrasound uses high-frequency sound waves to create images," he explained as he gently moved the probe (called a transducer) over the area. He moved the computer screen around so I could see the images. I intently watched the images as he moved back and forth and then in a circular motion. He passed over the nipple area and stopped briefly, moved to one side, then the other and again back to the nipple area. There it was...a distorted image sitting underneath my nipple. Then he was done.

"I'll have Karen take you back to the other room where you can get dressed," he stated flatly and left the room. There were no further explanations. I sat up and waited for Karen.

"You can get dressed now," she said as she ushered me back to the other room.

"Dr. Benjamen knows that you will be seeing Dr. Shorn this afternoon, so he will read your films immediately and send the results over to the office." She closed the door and left.

Hold it. That's it? But I have questions.

No, I really didn't. The truth was I didn't know what to think much less ask. I already knew the answer to the one question I didn't really want to ask anyway. I got dressed and left the room. Thank goodness there was no one in the waiting room. I was not in the mood to make any more small talk.

I had three hours before my next doctor's appointment. I went to my car and sat there. I didn't want to go back to work. I wasn't hungry. I didn't know what to do. I did notice that during the time I had been in the hospital, the car windows had frosted over. I started the car and turned the defroster on high. The air from the fan was as cold as the air outside. But I didn't notice it. I was void of thought. Slowly the defroster started to blow warm air. I continued just to sit there and watch the frost slowly melt away. I looked at the clock and realized that I had just been sitting there for over five minutes. I put the car in reverse and pulled out of the parking lot still unsure where to go. And then, like an epiphany, it became very clear.

I knew the one thing I didn't want to do was to talk to anyone, not even Leon. Although I did not have the official prognosis, I had a pretty strong inclination by the pit in my stomach that the results from the tests were not going to be very good. I needed some time alone to gather my thoughts and to gather strength to deal whatever the outcome turned out to be. I headed to the most logical place. I parked in front of my church.

"Dear God, we need to talk," I whispered as I entered through the side door. I could hear Pastor Poovey talking with someone in his office. I walked by as fast I could and hoped no one would see me. I went to the very front pew and sat down. It felt a little awkward at first because I usually don't sit that close to the front. I sat there with my head hung low, almost afraid to breathe. Finally I looked at the cross hanging above the altar. I just stared at it. I don't remember blinking. And then without warning I began to cry. I cried for me. I cried for the deep-seated fear I felt for the unknown. I cried selfishly because I did not want to die. I wanted to live, with my whole heart, I wanted to live. I wanted to see my children grow. I wanted to be there to watch them as they created their own lives. I wanted to go to places I hadn't been. I wanted to laugh more. I wanted to play more. I just wanted more time.

And then as quickly as the tears came, they subsided. And I began to pray. I prayed for forgiveness, for more time, for strength to fight "this thing," and a sign that He heard me. I really needed to know that He heard me. "Dear God, this me, Candace. Can you hear me? I'm in real trouble here. I need your help. Hey, are you there?"

I needed to know He was paying attention. I've read where people felt a presence or a light shined on them and I wanted to know that feeling. I needed to be reassured. I needed something, anything…to know that He had heard me. I wasn't just afraid. It was more than that. There was a penetrating fear deep in my soul that I was going to die.

But there was only quiet. I continued to sit there, hoping something miraculous would land on me and comfort me and tell me everything was going to be all right. But there was only quiet. I waited and waited, but the quiet lingered on.

I took a deep breath. *It's time to get on with it,* I thought, feeling a little dejected. It felt I had been there forever. I decided to go back to work and occupy some time before the next appointment at 2:00 p.m. There was no point in calling Leon. I didn't have anything to tell him yet.

* * * * * * * * * * * *

I checked out of the office for the day. I knew I wouldn't be up to coming back to work. The cold February wind whipped against my face as I walked to my car. It's funny because I hate the cold but I was oblivious to it today. I was a little preoccupied with the upcoming appointment. I arrived fifteen minutes early. I always arrive early. I was surprised to find the waiting room empty.

Well, that's good news, there aren't any sick people today...well except for me. But when I think about it, I don't feel sick either.

"Candace, you can come in," Betty said as she motioned to the door. The butterflies were having a hay-day in my stomach. "It's sure cold outside today," she said making small talk. "You can go to room three. Dr. Shorn will be in shortly."

Yeah, yeah, I've heard that before! I smiled and nodded okay.

It was a miracle, not necessarily the miracle I was hoping for, but Dr. Shorn entered the room before I had barely sat down. He had my folder—my future—in his hands. He opened it and placed on the desk.

"I have your mammogram and ultrasound reports from Dr. Benjamen. He called, and we discussed the results," he began as he thumbed through the paperwork. "There is a palpable suspicious mass in your right breast and a questionable mammographic lesion on the left side as well." I could feel the blood rush to my feet. I realized that I was holding my breath because my chest began hurting. I slowly exhaled.

"After our discussion, we feel that you need to have a biopsy as soon as possible." He looked at me intently. "The problem is…" he took a deep breath and carefully chose his words before he continued, "I am a part of this medical community and can only suggest this as an option after you have ruled out seeking treatment here. It is your choice, and I will abide by your decision to go to Billings for further tests. I understand that you want a second opinion. I am obligated to recommend an excellent surgeon who I know will take good care of you. Do you want me to call him to set up an appointment for you?"

"I want a second opinion and would prefer to have further tests in Billings. Can you recommend a good doctor?" I said hesitantly.

"Can you go anytime?" he asked as he started for the door.

"Yes, I'll make it work." I answered back, and he left the room. I sat there reflecting on the conversation. My heart raced a little when I replayed him saying, "suspicious mass," "lesion on left side," and "you should have a biopsy ASAP." The demons were having a heyday! I wanted them to stop!

Dr. Shorn returned and sat down. "I couldn't get who I had hoped for, but his associate was available, and he assured me that he was a fine surgeon also. His name is Dr. Hurie. Your appointment is for Monday afternoon at 3:30 p.m. at the Deaconess Clinic. Since it's a three- to three-and-a-half-hour drive to Billings, I scheduled it later in the afternoon so you wouldn't have to leave until the mid-morning on Monday and still have time to get there. I will send all the films with you so you don't have to have the x-rays repeated. I will fax my report to him so he has that also. Dr. Hurie will look the films over and then discuss what options are available to you. I would make plans to stay overnight. Do you have any questions?"

I looked at him and asked calmly, "Do I have cancer?"

"I don't know, but the mass in your right breast is very suspicious. Until you have a formal biopsy it cannot be confirmed. My concern is when you feel the mass, it does not move, and it is hard. Usually benign masses or fibrous tissues are flexible and will move slightly when pushed. The other concern I have is the size. It is a substantial mass. Additionally, when I checked the lymph node area, there was also suspicious involvement there. That's why I think it's imperative you have this taken care of immediately." He looked at me. "I wish I had better news. Do you have any other questions?"

I shook my head, no, and with that he left the room.

I left the doctor's office feeling numb. I headed home. Thoughts of suspicious mass, questionable lesion and lymph nodes kept my mind busy. It was hard to digest. I got home and headed straight for the bedroom. I took my shirt and bra off and took a really good look at myself in the mirror. I could not believe what I was seeing! I was horrified! My right breast was distorted. *Why haven't I noticed that before?* I raised my right arm and did an examination. Yes, it was still there—what did he say? "A palpable, suspicious mass?" *Whatever that means!* I slowly moved to the underarm area. My knees began to buckle under me. I grabbed for the edge of the dresser. I could not believe what I was feeling! *Get a hold of yourself, Candace,* I said to myself sternly. I took a deep breath. I stood up straight and again raised my right arm and began to feel along the armpit area. There it was—hard, protruding nodules. Not one but many. I put my arm down. I continued to stare at the mirror. "Oh, God, help me, please." I finally managed to say. I took one last look and got dressed again.

I sat in the living room and looked out the window. The cold north wind was blowing snow across the road causing a minor road blizzard. I shivered but not from the cold. What was happening to me? I didn't understand what was happening to me. The demons were drunk with joy.

"Dear Lord, please help me to be strong. I am afraid, and I am sorry that I am afraid. But God, I do not want to die. I do not know Your will, and I pray, Lord, that you give me courage to face whatever the outcome. I am trying to be strong. I want to be strong. I pray for your forgiveness, for your love, and for your understanding." I sat quietly. *Oh God, what am I going to do?* The echo of the second hand ticking away precious time penetrated by very being. I heard the furnace as it clunked and clinked, the pilot light igniting forcefully as it prepared itself to warm the house. And then like a blind man seeing for the first time. I focused on the issue at hand. *I want it out! I want it gone!* With renewed determination, I gathered what little strength I had and called Leon to let him know that we were headed to Billings.

* * * * * * * * * * * * *

"What are you going to tell the kids?" Leon asked as we were finalizing our road trip to Billings.

"I don't know. I suppose I will tell them what we know. I have a lump. It needs to be checked. We are going to Billings on Monday and returning on Tuesday. Everything will be fine.... Don't worry."

"Are you going to tell anyone else?"

"Well, I will have to tell my mother what's going on, because the kids will probably go over there for food. But I really don't want to worry her. What do you think I should tell her?"

"I guess the same as the kids. Are you going to tell them today or tomorrow?"

"Let's wait until tomorrow. You know what I would really like to do? I would like to go to church tomorrow (regardless of how I felt about my last visit. I needed the comfort I felt after I attended church.) Then we should go out for lunch like we normally do. After lunch I'll break the news that we are headed to Billings and why. Maybe if we don't make it a big deal no one will worry too much about it. I know," I added as an afterthought. "I'll tell them it is simply a precautionary measure."

"Are you going to tell the rest of the family? What about Ron and Judy, Rita and Larry, and 'the girls?'"

"No, I don't think I'll say anything yet. I don't have energy to answer questions I don't have the answers to. Let's just wait."

* * * * * * * * * * * * *

It had been overcast and cloudy all week and the temperature never got above 10 degrees below zero. Occasionally the north wind would come up causing drifts in the fields that reminded me of sand dunes, only white.

It was Sunday morning and finally the sun was shining. I have to admit it was beautiful. Everything looked so clean and untouched. Frost blanketed the trees and it was still cold. At least the sun gave you a false sense that it was warmer.

As was the normal routine on Sunday morning, Leon made breakfast. It was a family tradition passed down from his father. After breakfast we dressed for church as usual. We left for church twenty minutes early as usual. As was the custom we greeted everyone as we made our way to "our pew" to sit down. My mother and her two sisters were already there as usual. And as was the normal routine, the music started as Pastor Poovey walked down the aisle to the sanctuary as we sang the opening hymn. We stood for the opening and then sat down and followed along as the readings were recited. We stood for the gospel reading and as usual we sat down for the sermon.

Pastor Poovey moved to the pulpit. He looked at the congregation and as usual he began his sermon in a clear and strong voice.

He said, "In our gospel lesson this morning, St. John issues the call to eternal life to anybody who can read, anybody who can hear, or anybody who can see. He said this. 'Many are the signs Jesus did in the presence of his disciples, which are not written in this book, but these have been written that you might believe that Jesus is the Messiah, the Son of God, and that believing you might have life—through his name.'"

I know this wasn't necessarily new information but it caught my attention. *Did I hear him say something about believing and eternal life?* I sat up and listened intently.

"Life—we all want a life. But we want a life without hassles. We want a life without troubles. We want a life without pain. But folks, in the real world that's not going to happen. There is not going to be a life without hassles, without pain, without troubles this side of heaven. So what is life to be all about? St. John's book, the one we call the gospel of St. John in the Holy Bible, is, in its entirety, from beginning to end, about life. St. John says over and over again what life is to be about and even gives us the secret to life—life now, day in and day out, and life everlasting. He says simply, 'Life is about Jesus Christ.' Jesus Christ, the Son of God, is God's ultimate word to the world about life. John wanted people to know that Jesus came to us to issue a call for new life, the call of the new life that comes from believing in the death and resurrection of Jesus the Christ. John's gospel is full of human things that happened and human stories that Jesus told. They show people how Jesus was reaching out to touch the hearts of people with the good news of God. The good news that God loves and forgives no matter how hard-hearted people may be. The good news that he promises salvation—not by your works—you cannot earn your way into heaven, but he promises salvation by grace, by His love and His mercy."

Excuse me! I felt like there was a spotlight on me! Surely the sermon was written only for me. I looked around to see if everyone was looking at me! *No, those that weren't nodding off or disciplining their children were intently listening to the minister.*

"And he offers to all who turn to Him through the power of the Holy Spirit, eternal life. John recorded in his gospel through the power of the Holy Spirit, Jesus' very words. Jesus said, 'I am the life of the world. I am the bread of life.' John tells us over and over again that Jesus offers life, and he offers not only plain, simple vanilla life, but he offers an abundant life. As you and I hear that, we also hear and understand that an abundant life is not necessarily a life with more material possessions. When we have an abundant life in Christ that does not mean that we are going to be healthier."

Does Pastor Poovey know...how could he know? Leon is the only one who knows except the doctor and nurse and they're bound by their oath not to tell anyone. I felt flushed. My palms were sweaty.

"That is not the promised life that Jesus said he would give us. Jesus never promised that following Him would make life easier. In fact, in may get harder. Jesus never promised that following Him, we would never have any troubles; the fact is we may have more troubles."

The tears welled up in my eyes. I struggled not to let them fall. I couldn't believe what I was hearing!

"He does say that when you trust in Him as your personal Savior, your life is linked with Him, with God the Father, with God the Son, and with God the Holy Spirit. Whatever your troubles, whatever your problems, whatever is coming down on you, I am here to tell you that God is with you."

At that very moment I wanted to shout at the top of my lungs, "Praise you Lord, and thank you God!" I wanted to run down the aisle and give that minister a big kiss on the cheek! I was ecstatic with joy and could hardly contain myself!

"He loves you. He will not forsake you, and He can give you the ability to get through whatever is coming down on you. He's not going to take it away. But knowing how much God loves us gives us the only true security there is in life. In Jesus' name, amen."

I was amazed. I felt jubilant and yet exhausted. He had heard my prayer! Yes, God had answered my prayer. It was my miracle!

Pastor Poovey could have talked about anything that Sunday. He could have preached about sin, about people who don't go to church, about forgiveness, about anything else, but he talked about life, everlasting life. He talked about life not always going to be easy or turn out the way we wanted it to be. I got the message. I left the church with renewed hope. I was still unsure about my future but I knew that I was in good hands. Don't get me wrong, I continued to feel afraid but it was different now. I felt I had courage to face whatever the outcome. I had determination and was ready to fight the fight because I knew that God was with me, that He had not forsaken me. My faith was reaffirmed.

When I think back and when I am not blindsided with my troubles, I know that God has always been there for me. I had just lost sight of that for the moment.

We left the church and headed out for lunch. On the way we stopped by the grocery store to pick up the Sunday paper. On the front page the feature story was, "Surviving Cancer." It's true. I'm serious. God is good, very, very good.

The unthankful heart…discovers no mercies; but the thankful heart…will find, in every hour some heavenly blessings.

—Henry Ward Beecher

Chapter Four
Get Rid of Anything That Isn't Useful, Beautiful, or Joyful

Everyone took the news quite well. I assured them this was simply a precautionary measure and there was nothing to worry about. My mother was going to have the children come over Monday night for supper. I envied them, she was the great cook!

Leon loaded the luggage into the car. It was time to go. We wanted to leave a little early just in case there were some icy spots along the way.

"Are you ready?" he asked.

"I was born ready!" I said with faked enthusiasm. I kept replaying Dr. Shorn's concerns over and over in my mind. *The demons kept reappearing!* I could not fathom the thought of me having cancer. My self-talk was damaging my resolve to be strong, to be able to conquer anything I was going to be up against. I was reverting back to feeling afraid. How quickly a person becomes weak again!

"Well, it's off to see the doctor," I sang to the tune of "We're off to See the Wizard," or at least I tried. Trust me, I cannot carry a tune! "It's off to see the doctor—because of the things he duz." The words didn't quite fit the tune. But it didn't matter much that it wasn't making sense. None of this was making much sense. I smiled at him.

I hadn't told Leon the whole story yet. He knew about the lump in my right breast, but I failed to mention the suspicious lesion in the left breast and the numerous lymph nodes that were sticking out from under my arm. My first instinct was to protect those I care about. The one lump was enough for him to worry about for the time being. I figured he didn't need to know there was more—a lot more.

Oh, my dear Leon, this is going to get interesting. I hope you are ready. I have a feeling I am going to be leaning on you a lot before this is all said and done.

* * * * * * * * * * * * *

It was a bright sunny Monday morning. The snow glistened in the sun. The trees were white with frost. The day had a certain "Currier and Ives" feel to it minus the horses and sleighs, minus the pine trees, minus the…oh well, you get the picture!

"Let's get this show on the road," I said as I watched him put on his winter coat. Leon had started the car earlier, and it was nice and toasty inside. We headed down the road listening to the radio, both lost in our own thoughts.

"What do you want to do for Valentine's Day?" he asked out of the blue.

"I don't know. I haven't thought about it. When is the fourteenth?"

"I think it's this Wednesday or Thursday. I thought it would be nice if we went out for supper. Steak and lobster sound good, don't you think?"

"It's been a long time since we had steak and lobster. It does sound good." We got quiet again.

"You know this might be a good time to quit smoking—for good this time." I announced as I lit a cigarette and cracked a window so the smoke could escape. I looked at it and laughed. What an oxymoron!

Leon looked at me and smiled. "I agree. It's time to quit." We continued to make small talk off and on throughout the three-and-a-half-hour drive. The roads were clear most of the way, and we arrived in Billings early, as usual.

"Let's do a little shopping. Let's go to the lumber yard. You know we have been talking about remodeling the bathroom. We could see what they have for showers and that kind of stuff." This set the stage for the rest our conversation. We spent the next hour or so checking out things we thought would be great for the new bathroom. We made all sorts of plans. It was fun. But time was up, and it was time for my doctor's appointment.

The doctor's office was located on the other side of town, about a twenty to thirty minute drive depending on traffic. We had been to Billings many times so we were familiar with the city. As we made our way across town, we talked a little more about the remodel. Again we got absorbed in our own thoughts.

"Leon, what if he tells me I have cancer and that I am dying?" I asked. The question surprised even me!

He glanced over at me and then turned his attention back to the road and the city traffic. He didn't say a word. I kept looking at him waiting for his response. He kept his eyes on the road. I slowly turned my head and looked out the window. I didn't ask the question again. It wasn't worth repeating. I guess we both thought if we didn't talk about it, we wouldn't have to deal with it. I think it was Scarlett O'Hara from *Gone with the Wind* who said, "I won't think about it today. I'll think about it tomorrow." There is much to be said about denial.

* * * * * * * * * * * * *

The cold north wind hit us square in the face as we made our way across the clinic parking lot. I remembered how much I hated the cold as it seemed to penetrate right through my winter coat. I clung onto Leon's arm. I wasn't sure if it was for protection against the wind or support for what lay ahead. My appointment with Dr. Hurie was at 3:30 p.m. His office was located on the second floor and we arrived early as usual. Once more I had to fill out paperwork. It was almost identical to the form I had filled out in Glendive and of course it was front and back. It was easier this time because I knew all the answers to the questions. I handed the completed form and my films to the receptionist. We took our seats and waited. We said very little and continued to ignore the question I had asked earlier.

"Candace Eide," the nurse called.

I rose from my chair. "I'll be back in a second." I said as I obediently followed the nurse. We stopped by the scale, and she weighed me, still 145.

"I'll have you go to room two," she said. She took my blood pressure, pulse, temperature…and a gown. "Take everything off except your underwear and socks. I gave Dr. Hurie your films. He will be in shortly," she said and left the room.

I undressed and skillfully put the gown on. *I am now master of the gown!* I looked for a magazine to thumb through. I needed something to occupy my thoughts. The demons were getting ready to pounce. I waited for the doctor to come in. I hate waiting.

Dr. Hurie entered. He was small in stature, about five feet six inches. He had short black, wavy hair that reminded me of my brother's hair. I was always envious of my brother's hair. It was thick, black and had natural waves. It cost me about thirty-five dollars to get my waves.

Dr. Hurie extended his hand. "Hi, I am Dr. Hurie," he said. He had a warm smile and a confident hand shake. He started with trivial questions about the weather and the roads and finally got to the problem at hand.

"I'll have you come over here," he said as pointed to the exam table. He repeated the same procedure Dr. Shorn had done in Glendive. You would think that exposing myself three times in a week, it would get easier. But you'd be wrong. He gently guided me upright.

"I looked at your films." He took a breath and continued. "Dr. Shorn also faxed me his reports. There is a concern about a spot on your left breast that needs further investigation. I want you to have another mammogram to compare it with this one. I will have the nurse make an appointment for you." And then he looked me straight in the eyes and said. "I would like to schedule you for surgery. I can do it this Thursday if that works for you. It would save you a trip back to Glendive."

"Surgery? Already on Thursday?" I asked, very surprised!

"After looking at the films and reading Dr. Shorn's and Dr. Benjamen's reports, I agree that a biopsy is necessary. A biopsy will require surgery." He went on to explain. "First you will be placed under general anesthesia. I will do a lumpectomy, which is the removal of the affected area. It will be taken down to the lab, frozen, and then tested. This process takes about two hours. Once I have the results back one of two things will happen. Either I will close up the incision or do a modified radical mastectomy. The modified radical mastectomy procedure requires the removal of the entire breast, the entire breast tissue, including the nipple and the areola (the pigmented skin around the nipple) and most of the lymph nodes in the armpit. There will be a six-to-eight-inch incision." He stopped to take a breath. "Do you think you will want to have reconstruction?"

The truth is I heard or understood very little of what he said. My head was spinning. I just kept staring at him.

"I guess you can make that decision later. I will leave what is called a flap, should you decide to have reconstruction later."

"You want to do surgery this Thursday?" I asked, trying to absorb the information he had given me.

He noticed my dazed look. "Yes, I would like to do surgery on Thursday," he said gently. "Since you are already in Billings it would save you a trip back to Glendive. My other concern is, if I don't schedule it for this Thursday it will be two weeks or possibly more before I can do it. I would rather not wait that long. Will Thursday be a problem?"

"Ah, I guess Thursday is okay. I didn't think it would happen this quickly," I answered back. "Can I talk it over with my husband to make sure it works for him?"

"Absolutely, and in the meantime I will schedule a mammogram for you. One other thing, don't let anyone have these films. Keep them with you." He smiled. "Lately, for some reason, it seems films get lost between here and crossing the street to the hospital." He stood and left the room, leaving me alone, just sitting there in that stupid gown.

Wow. In a week's time I had found a lump, discovered there were many lumps, and now a surgery to get rid of at least one of my breasts was being planned. This was moving fast. I hardly had time to think, except for the demons. There was a soft tap on the door as it opened, and Dr. Hurie's nurse entered.

"I have scheduled your mammogram for tomorrow morning at 9:00 a.m. Will that work?" she asked.

"I suppose so," I answered back, still in a daze.

"Dr. Hurie said you wanted to talk to your husband. While you are getting dressed I will go get him and have him come back here. And I'll take these," she said as she grabbed the large manila envelope with my x-rays in it. I started to say no because Dr. Hurie had told me to hang on to them. At *least I think that is what he said.* But it was fuzzy. She was Dr. Hurie's nurse, so he must want to look at them again. I said nothing. I gathered myself together, dressed, and waited for Leon.

He carefully opened the door and peeked in.

"Come in," I said. "Have a seat." I took a deep breath. "Hey, there is a plan. I have a mammogram scheduled for tomorrow. There is a spot on my left breast he wants to check out."

Leon looked a little surprised.

"It gets better." I didn't pause as he frowned over the information about my left breast. "He wants to do surgery this Thursday. It's the only opening he has for two weeks, maybe longer, plus it would save us a trip back to Glendive and then back here again."

Leon looked at me. "Okay," he said slowly. He was still frowning.

"Will it be a problem for you to get off work?"

"Things are pretty slow right now with it being so cold. I guess it will work."

"It's happening pretty quickly, don't you think?" I said as I watched for a sign that he wasn't sure about all this.

"Is it cancer?" he asked.

"They don't know yet. He has to do a biopsy. I think he said something about opening up the breast, taking a sample, something about freezing it, testing it for cancer, then doing either a lumpectomy or a modified radical mastectomy, depending on the results from the test. Oh, and he said something about waiting two hours. But I can't remember what that was about, though."

"You said there is a spot on your left side also?" he was asking when Dr. Hurie entered the room.

"Hi, I'm Dr. Hurie," he said as he extended his hand to Leon. Leon took it and introduced himself. "Did you decide if Thursday was okay?"

"Guess so."

"Good. I will have you come in Wednesday afternoon. Bring your films with you, and we can compare the results with your other mammogram."

I looked at him quite puzzled. "Your nurse took my films. I assumed you wanted to look at them again."

"But I told you…" and he stopped. "That's okay. I won't need to see you on Wednesday. I will see you on Thursday before surgery. I'll have a nurse bring you information on what you need to do before surgery." He stood up to leave, "Candace and Leon, enjoy your stay. Go out and have a nice dinner." He extended his hand and shook ours. "Have faith; things are going to be fine." He left the room. We left the clinic.

* * * * * * * * * * * *

We had made a motel reservation, but it was only for one night. We were staying at a motel located across the street from the clinic and hospital. It was a nice place and definitely convenient. When we checked in we extended the reservation for five days. We figured we would be there at least that long, although we weren't sure how long I would be in the hospital after surgery. We were lucky. They gave special rates for families who had someone in the hospital.

"I suppose we'd better call the kids and my mother and let them know we are staying longer than we thought," I said, dreading the call. "I guess we should call everyone and let them know I am having surgery. And then I suppose we should go shopping. I didn't bring a housecoat. I am sure you are going to need underwear and socks. I know I didn't bring enough underwear. Do you have enough shirts?

What about pants? Maybe we should go home and come back a little better prepared," I rambled on, almost in a panic.

"Candace," Leon said softly, "we can pick up a few items. I'm sure they have a washer and dryer. I can do a load of clothes if I need to. It will be okay."

Have faith; it will be okay. These are fine platitudes to give someone, but when you are the receiver and scared out of your wits it doesn't seem to lighten the worry. I was confused as to what was happening. I heard the words the doctor said, but I was having a problem comprehending the meaning of it all.

"Let's go have a nice dinner, and then when we get back we'll call everyone and let them know what's happening."

It sounded like a good plan, and I relaxed a little. There was a small dilemma. I wasn't very hungry. But I did need a diversion. The demons wanted to party. We cleaned up and went searching for a nice place to eat. As we drove I silently prayed, *Dear God, I pray that I have the courage to deal with what lies ahead. I pray, Lord, for strength to keep the demons at bay. And God, thank you for Leon. I know that you are my Savior and my rock to stand on, but I thank you for Leon. He is my shoulder to lean on.*

* * * * * * * * * * * * *

It had been a long time since just the two of us had gone on a trip by ourselves. All our other travels included camping trips or holidays with family. We spent the next three days enjoying each other's company. I had managed to put the demons to rest, at least for the moment.

Leon was an early riser, so every morning he would get up, get the paper, and bring back cups of hot coffee. After we read the paper, we dressed and would go out for a late breakfast. The first day I spent most it on the phone calling everyone and answering the same questions over and over again. Then we walked over to the hospital to find out where I needed to go Thursday morning. We spent the next day walking through the malls (there were two), and the last day we went to an afternoon matinee. Each evening we went out for a nice dinner. It was quite enjoyable. I had almost forgotten why we were really there.

We finally decided this would be a good time to quit smoking. I had always heard the first three days of quitting were the hardest. In all my efforts before I had never gone that long! The truth is I don't think I ever made it through a half day before I was searching for a half-smoked butt—that certainly is an appropriate term—much less three days! I figured I would be in the hospital that long, and since I couldn't smoke there, it was a perfect time.

Our last night before surgery was Wednesday, February 14. As we had discussed on our way up, we had steak and lobster, although the initial plan didn't include dinner out in Billings! We ate early. I wasn't supposed to have anything after 10:00 p.m. But I wanted to play it really safe. I didn't want to eat anything after 7:00 p.m.

After dinner we decided to try our luck and went to a casino. It was a little after 7:00 and we hoped our money would last us at least until 9:00 p.m. We each had $10.00! We are the last of the big spenders! After an hour or so I had began getting a little antsy. I was ready to go. It was unusual because I liked to gamble, but a demon would pop up suddenly and maliciously remind me what lay ahead tomorrow. Plus, I was getting down to my last nickel. At the same time Leon found me, his $10.00 spent. I lit what I hoped would be my last cigarette. As we walked toward the door I noticed a gal lighting one up. I walked over to her and handed her my cigarette lighter and case and said, "I've decided to quit," and we walked out the door.

True to our resolve, Leon and I have never smoked again. I always thought when I did quit smoking it would be a time of celebration. But the truth is I never thought about it again. I sometimes feel a twinge of guilt that I gave my cigarettes away instead of throwing them away, but at the time cigarettes still had value.

* * * * * * * * * * * *

The day of reckoning finally arrived. It was Thursday morning, February 15. Did I get any sleep? No, not very much. Was I nervous? Yes, butterflies were flitting everywhere. Was I afraid? Actually I was not afraid. I think there is a difference between being nervous and being afraid. I wasn't afraid of the surgery. But I was nervous about the outcome. I think it's a bit like a performer who goes on stage. They are not afraid to go on stage but are nervous waiting for the show to begin. I was very nervous waiting for the show to begin!

It was still dark outside when we left the motel to walk across the street to the hospital. And though it was cold it had warmed up considerably...it was zero degrees and there was no wind! *It was a virtual heat wave!* I clung to Leon's arm for support. We didn't say a word. We knew where we were going, why we were going there and what was going to happen when we got there! Finally or at least this time there were no surprises. And yes, we arrived early!

I checked in at the desk. It didn't take long and the nurse called me to follow her. She indicated that Leon could come too. We obeyed.

"You can get undressed and put your belongings into this bag," she said. "If you have any valuables like a watch or rings, I suggest giving them to your husband." I didn't have anything. I had left everything in the room just like the brochure had suggested. "When you are finished you can get into bed. While you are waiting please fill out this form. I will be back in a minute," she said as she handed me the clipboard. *Are you serious? Another form? The clinic is right across the street! Can't you people share information?* I was a little annoyed that I had to complete yet another form.

I undressed and put my clothes in the bag. The last thing I wanted to do was get into bed. I held the clipboard and answered the same questions again...for the third time! When I was through I started pacing back and forth. Leon sat quietly in a chair. There really wasn't much to say. The nurse finally returned.

"Okay, let's get started," she said as she motioned me to get into bed. She took my temperature, pulse, and blood pressure. She picked up the clipboard and fired question after question. Obviously she had done this many, many times before. "When did you eat and drink last? Have you had a bowel movement today?"

I wonder why she needed to know that?

"Do you smoke? Do you have any known allergies? Who do I contact in case of an emergency?" Then she went over the consent form and the form where they are not responsible for anything that goes wrong. And last but not least, requested that I sign on the dotted line indicating that I had read and understood everything she had just gone over with me.

I wonder what would happen if I refused to sign. Would they not do the surgery? What were my options? To sign a form they created to protect themselves and have the surgery, or not sign the form and they refuse the surgery? It was just a question. I signed the form.

"I think that will do for now. Are you warm enough? She asked. "We have heated blankets if you would like one."

"Yes, that would be nice," I answered. I suddenly realized that I was cold. I hate being cold. She left and soon returned with a warm blanket. It felt wonderful. *Finally someone discovered "heat" and got it right!* The nurse had barely left the room when another person walked in. It was the anesthesiologist. He had a clipboard in his hand. *You've got to be kidding? Not another form!*

"Hi, I am Dr. Theo," he said. "I will be administering the anesthesia. It's my job to make sure you don't feel a thing." He smiled and then he asked, "Are you a smoker?"

"I was a smoker," I said.

"How long have you quit smoking?" He asked

"Last night around 9:00," I answered. I was blushing. I could feel the blood rushing to my cheeks. I was embarrassed. It was first time I was really felt ashamed that I had to admit that I was a smoker.

He tilted his head to the side and smiled again. "Well, I am glad that you have quit! But I will take precautionary measures because your lungs haven't had time to adjust yet. People who smoke have a greater risk of phenomena after surgery. I will do whatever I can to make sure that it doesn't happen." He wrote a few notes and then he went over the procedure. "Do you have any questions?"

I shook my head no. I had no questions. *How could I have questions when I couldn't absorb the information they were giving me? It seemed like I would latch onto one thing, and the rest was lost to me. And when I thought I got it all, those damn demons would interfere. I was just doing what I was told. It was all getting frustrating.*

He smiled and patted my hand. "We'll see you in a few minutes," he said and then he left. Leon and I sat in quiet.

"You should go have breakfast while I'm in surgery," I said, breaking the silence. "I will be in there for a while."

"I'll see" he answered back. "Right now I'm not very hungry. How are you doing?"

"I don't know." I sighed. The demons were dancing with excitement. They were devising evil plots. According to their plan I was going to sleep for a long, long time. "You know Leon, I still can't believe I am lying in this bed waiting to see if I am going to wake up with one breast or two. None of this makes sense. I wish this was over, to tell you the truth."

"I know. I wish there was something I could do," he said as he got up and moved closer to the bed. He gently held my hand. "You know that you are going to be okay. Everything is going to be okay."

"Yeah, I know. I just wish it was over," I answered just as Dr. Hurie entered the room.

"Good morning," he said, smiling.

At least he looks rested!

"Good morning," Leon and I said at the same time.

"I want to go over the procedure one more time with you and answer any questions if you have any," he said as he picked up the clipboard at the end of the bed and thumbed through it. He repeated the information he had given me in his office. My heart was racing! Finally he finished with, "The whole operation will take about four to five hours."

Oh God, I can't believe this is happening!

He looked at me searching for a sign that I understood what he was saying.

In a few hours a part of me, a part that identifies me as a woman will most likely be gone. I will never be the same. Please, Lord, give me the strength to survive this. I am sorry. I am trying to be strong. I am trying to trust you that everything is going to be all right. But Lord, I am afraid. I still can't believe this is happening to me. I don't understand. I just lay there with a sheepish grin on my face, nodding as if I heard every word he said. He turned to Leon.

"Leon, the nurse will take you to the waiting room. You will check in with the receptionist, and then you can leave if you want to. When you leave the receptionist will ask where you can be reached just in case." He smiled. "Do either of you have any questions?"

Neither one of us had anything to say.

"Okay." He turned to go and then stopped. He turned back to me and said, "Candace, I believe God only gives you what you can handle. You are going to be fine." And then he left. Leon and I looked at each other. We were both stunned by that remark. I bowed my head and prayed softly, "Thank you, God, for loving me. Please forgive me for my weakness. I do trust in You."

The curtain was pushed open. "It's time to go. Are you ready?" the nurse said as she grabbed the clipboard from the bedside table and put in on the end of the bed. *She is much too cheerful!* She unlocked the legs of the bed and started out of the room. "I love you," I managed to say as she started to wheel me down to surgery.

"But we just met!" she quipped and then she laughed. I was slightly caught off-guard by her response, and then I laughed also. She stopped.

Leon had a confused look on his face and then he finally got it too. He smiled. He walked over and kissed me on the forehead and softly whispered, "I love you, too."

What a wonderful thing to do. I know that not everyone would have appreciated it, but I was grateful the nurse had the forethought to lighten the mood. It did make me feel better. It was time to get this

"thing" out of my body. It was time to get my life back on track. *Dear God, please guide Dr. Hurie's hands. I pray that it all goes well. And thank you, God, for being with me.*
The temperature from the hall to the operating room changed drastically. It was cold. I hate being cold. I shivered. No one noticed. The room was busy with activity. Surgical nurses were busy preparing the operating instruments. Everyone was in a very good mood. *Well, at least everyone seems to be happy. Don't want anyone taking their bad mood out on me!* The nurse moved the bed next to one that was situated under a big light. Everyone stopped what they were doing and focused their attention on me.

"Okay, on the count of three we are going to lift you and put on this bed," one of the nurses informed me. "One, two, three." I was quickly deposited on the other bed.

"See you later," the nurse who had delivered me said as she wheeled the other bed out.

"Hi, Candace, how are you doing?" One nursed asked as she checked my chart and hospital wristband. "I am going to start your IV, and then we'll prep the area Dr. Hurie will be working on," she said as she slipped a blood pressure cuff around my arm and then placed an oxygen tube into my nostrils.

I just smiled. I didn't have anything clever to say. I didn't have anything to say! I figured this was not a social event. Plus, I was not elated with joy to be there.

"Dr. Hurie and Dr. Theo should be arriving soon," she said as she began the IV. "There will be a little poke," she continued as she stuck the needle through my skin on top of my hand. I didn't flinch. I was so proud. She started the IV. Dr. Theo entered the operating room.

"Are you ready to get this done?" he asked as he tied a rubber strap around my arm. I smiled and nodded. He slightly flicked my vein with his finger. "Ah, that's a good, healthy one. You have excellent veins," he said as he slid a larger needle into the protruding vein. I watched intently. I discovered if I could see what was coming I didn't move. I hate surprises.

Dr. Hurie entered and greeted everyone. "Good news, Candace," he announced. "The picture that you had taken on Tuesday didn't show anything unusual. So I won't have to do anything with the left breast."

"Good," was all I could muster.

"Dr. Theo will start the anesthesia, and when you are ready, I will begin." He patted my shoulder. "We will take good care of you, Candace." I smiled and nodded. I could feel the anesthesia move through my vein.

"Slowly count backward starting at 100." Dr. Theo instructed.

"100, 99, 98, 97, 96, 95, 94, 93, 92…"

* * * * * * * * * * * * *

I struggled to open my eyes. People wearing white clothing were walking around, and I could hear a slow but steady, "beep, beep, beep," in the distance. I blinked. I was disoriented. I didn't know where I was. I wanted to go back to sleep. I closed my eyes.

"Good afternoon, Candace," someone said.

I opened my eyes again, and this time I recognized that the people in white were nurses. "It's time to wake up," she said cheerfully.

But I don't want to wake up. I want to go back to sleep. So just take your silly self and go away.

"Everything is looking good. It's time to get you to your room. I'm sure your husband is anxious to see you. I'll be right back with your things."

I watched as she walked away. The fuzziness was leaving. I remembered everything. I looked down at my chest. I wonder if I have one breast or two? I slowly lifted the blanket away and pulled the gown up at the neckline. My heart was pounding. But all I could see was bandages, tubes and brown gunk everywhere. The good news was I wasn't feeling any pain! But that didn't mean anything! I suppose the anesthesia was still working.

"Okay, I think I have everything," she said as unlocked the legs on the bed and began wheeling me to the room. "Your husband will be able to visit in a few minutes."

"Do I have one breast or two?" I asked.

"The doctor will be up to see you soon," was all that she said. I nodded.

I guess that means I only have one. Well, at least the cancer is gone, and it is done. I can get on with my life, I thought with renewed hope. What is that saying? Oh yeah, I remember. "If I only knew then what I know now!"

⊷══◉ ◉══⊷

The will of God will not take you where the grace of God cannot keep you.

—Anonymous

Chapter Five
There's No Place Like Home, There's No Place Like Home

The next three days were a blur. I was fortunate in that I had a double room and did not have a roommate. I was grateful for that. Dr. Theo was the first to come and see me. He reassured me that I handled everything very well and my lungs sounded fine. Dr. Hurie came in to see me a couple hours later. He gave me the news. I had cancer, and he had done a radical mastectomy. In other words, I was one breast short of a complete pair! It was official now. I think I handled the news rather well. But what a whirlwind ride this has been! In a short period of time—ten days to be exact—I found a lump, no many, many lumps, had my breasts examined more times than I thought imaginable and last but certainly not least, had a breast removed. Thank goodness it was over! Thank goodness I was still alive.

The realization I had only one breast had not sunk in yet. My entire chest area was covered in bandages. I was given strict orders that I could not shower or remove the bandages until Saturday. Dr. Hurie did say that on Saturday I could take a shower and if everything looked okay I could go home on Sunday. I wasn't going to do anything that would jeopardize that possibility.

Besides the bandages I had two tubes protruding through a hole in my skin. At the end of each tube was a bottle commonly referred to as a drain. It was shaped liked a hand grenade. One was attached just below the armpit area and the other attached to my tummy, about four inches below the incision. I had instructions to empty the bottles at least three times a day and log the amount of liquid in each and time of day I emptied them. Most of the time, the liquid had a cloudy, yellowish hue to it. Sometimes there was what looked like strings of blood floating around in it.

I was hooked up with an IV that contained a pain killer. All I had to do was push a little button and a dose would be released into my vein. If I needed I could give myself a dose every hour. But I decided that unless it was absolutely unbearable, I would not take advantage of the new technology in medicine. The good news was I did not have a lot of pain…unless I tried to lift my right arm! *Wow! You didn't have to hit me twice! I tried raising my arm once, and that was enough for me.*

There was a great deal of discomfort when I tried to reach out or raise my right arm. I knew it would be a problem later because I was right-handed, but at the moment I didn't have to deal with the issue. I was sure it hurt because of the surgery, but why did it hurt so much under the armpit? The demons were starting to play their tricks again! I shook them off. *I'm sure everything will be just fine in a week or two,* I told myself with fake confidence. I surprised myself at how well I was able to manage everything I needed to do at this point with my left arm.

Leon arrived every morning around 10:00 a.m. By that time I had eaten, gotten my sponge bath, and the bed had been changed. We would spend part of the day walking around the hospital—dragging the IV machine with us—and the other part watching TV.

I was taken aback at my reaction the first time we went for a walk. I held my right arm close to my body. Initially I thought it was because it was more comfortable, but then I realized that I did it to cover the fact I was flat-chested on one side, and someone might notice it. I was embarrassed. *For goodness sakes, Candace, get yourself together. Who cares if you have one breast or two? Dang it demons, go away and leave me alone!*

Saturday finally arrived and I was going to take a shower! I was so relieved! I usually showered every day unless we went camping. And even then on the second day I at least washed my hair. Come to think of it, I don't ever remember Leon saying, "Good morning, beautiful." Generally he simply states, "You must have slept well!"

The truth is I can scare people in the morning with my morning look! I sometimes frighten myself! And it was going on three days since I had a shower or bath. But for all my excitement, was I ready for the unveiling? I wasn't sure if I was ready to look at what I was going to see? It will be the first time I will see myself with one breast.

It's no big deal. So you have one breast. You know that it doesn't make you less of a woman. The important thing to remember is the cancer is gone, and soon, very soon, you can go home and forget all about this. Focus on what is really important, not on something that has no value.

I was steadfast in my belief that it was going look just fine. Years ago I had worked in a nursing home, and one of the woman patients had had a mastectomy, and it didn't look so bad, although I had to admit it was kind of odd to see it the first time. But I am a grown woman with enough confidence to know that boobs do not make the woman, just like muscles do not make the man.

You keep telling yourself that and maybe soon you will believe it!

It was almost 8:30 a.m. I had eaten breakfast and was anxiously waiting for Dr. Hurie to do his morning rounds. The butterflies in my stomach were flitting about. I was nervous.

"Good morning, Candace," he said with his usual casual air and smile as he entered the room. He thumbed through my chart. "I guess today is the day we take off the bandages."

"And a shower. You said I could take a shower when the bandages came off," I replied.

"Yes, you can take a shower." He looked up from reading the notes.

The way he's looking at me, he's probably thinking, "Lady, you need a shower!"

"The notes state that you are taking very little medicine for the pain. It's there for you so you don't have to be in pain. Is there a problem that I am not aware of?" he asked.

"No, there is no problem. I am doing fine. What pain I have is tolerable. I have had worse," I answered back.

"Okay, but don't hesitate to use it if you need to. I'll have you sit on the edge of the bed," he said as he closed the door to my room. He unloosened the little clamp that held the bandages in place and slowly began to unwrap it.

"You'll have to raise your right arm," he said as he grabbed it and raised it up. I grimaced. "You will feel some tightness for a while. There are some exercises that you can do to help with that. I will have one of the nurses give you the information," he said as he continued to undo the bandage, taking care not to pull too much around the tubes that were protruding from body.

I could feel the blood leave my head. I felt flushed. I couldn't imagine what it was going to look like.

Oh God, please don't let it be hideous. Please give me the strength to bear what I am going to see.

Finally the last of the bandages were off. Dr Hurie continued his examination. He was saying something about a flap, stitches, drain tubes and treatment, but I didn't hear a word. I was too engrossed in what I was about to see. I slowly looked down. And there it was, or should I say, it wasn't. Where I once had a size B+—was nothing. In its place was an incision held together with staples. The surgical area was still covered with the brownish betadine solution. It definitely wasn't pretty, but surprisingly, it was okay.

Just be grateful it is over. You may only have one boob, but the cancer is gone.

"It looks really good," Dr Hurie said breaking into my thoughts. "Everything looks fine. When you take your shower make sure that you wash around the area. I'll have a nurse bring in an antibiotic for you to put on when you are done bathing. It looks like you are on track to go home tomorrow."

I pulled my hospital gown back up. "I am looking forward to that," I answered. "Will I be able to leave in the morning?"

"I'll try to be up here around the same time for one more checkup. Then you can go."

"Thank you. I really appreciate that."

"I'll see tomorrow," he said as he left the room.

I got up from the bed and closed the door. I wanted a better view. I turned towards the mirror. *Are you really ready for this? I pray for strength, Lord. I pray for courage to accept what I cannot change.* I took a deep breath as I slowly raised my gown. *The demons were at bay, but my emotions were running amok.* I stared at myself for a moment. There were no thoughts. I just kept looking. It wasn't registering in my mind that the person I was looking at in the mirror was me. It couldn't be me. The person I was looking at only had one breast. The person I was looking at had two red, puffy, gross-looking pieces of skin held together where the other breast should be. The person that I was seeing wanted to scream, "Why me?" The person I was looking at was appalled at what she was looking at! The person in the mirror had sad eyes. The person in the mirror just couldn't be me. *Oh please, God, I don't want it to be me.*

But the person in the mirror was me. I was different. I reached up with my left hand and gently touched the disfigured area. It was tender to the touch. I looked back at my reflection in the mirror, hoping I guess if I stared long enough things would go back to the way they were. But it didn't change.

"Okay, Candace, you have two choices. You can feel sorry for yourself or get on with the business of living." I said out loud to the person in the mirror. "You can decide right here and now, this very moment, to accept what you cannot change and make the best of it, or you can feel sorry for yourself and shrivel up and die. What do you want to do?"

I stared at myself for what seemed like an eternity. I was searching for that person who was usually cheerful and happy. I was looking for a sign that the person whose brother fondly called her "bright-eyes" still existed. I tilted my head to the left and then to the right. I leaned in for a closer look.

"Oh there you are." I managed to smile at the reflection in the mirror. I took a deep breath and stood up straight. "I choose to live," I said confidently. "I choose to live."

* * * * * * * * * * * * *

The shower felt great, although I had a challenge washing my hair with my left hand! I continued to favor my right arm. It was also a little disconcerting that when I looked down I could see my feet without any obstruction. And it was difficult to maneuver around the IV and tubes that were still attached to me. The biggest challenge was to wrap the towel around my head after the shower. I finally had to bite the bullet and use my right arm. I have to admit that I didn't waste any time to push the button for pain relief. But all in all I felt like a new person when I was finished. I reassured myself, "This, too, shall pass," and everything will be fine soon. This was my last day in the hospital. *I can put up with a few minor inconveniences for one more day.*

I was in a fresh gown, sitting on a chair when Leon arrived. "I see you got your shower finally." Leon said,

"Yeah, and I feel like a million bucks!" I said excitedly. And I meant it. After I made the decision to quit feeling sorry for myself and get on with living I felt invincible. *I have one boob, but I can live with that. The cancer is gone, and that's the most important thing.*

"Good news," I continued. "I get to go home tomorrow. Dr. Hurie said he will try to get up here as early as possible, and then we can go. I can hardly wait!"

"When will they take out the IV and drains?"

"I am assuming tomorrow. I really don't know. I never asked." *Let's see...what is that saying about "assume"? Oh, yeah, when you* assume *it is making an ass out of you and me! How quickly one forgets!*

"What's the weather like outside?" I asked.

"It's not too bad really. It's about 10 degrees, and according to the weather report it should stay like that at least until the end of the week."

"Hey, a regular heat wave out there!" I smiled. It didn't matter what the temperature was outside. Nothing could ruin my good mood. I was going home. I was going to get my normal life back. I could hardly wait.

Leon and I spent the rest of day just like we had spent the others. We went for a walk and then watched TV. The day was excruciatingly long. I was getting antsy and I wanted out. Finally day turned into night. Leon said his goodbyes and I laid in bed restless waiting for time to pass. The night was as long as the day. I thought it would never end. But finally morning came. And just like the days before, an aide brought me breakfast, I ate, then she came and got the tray. I took another shower. It was as good as the one yesterday. I was getting pretty good at using my left hand. I brushed my teeth and waited for Dr. Hurie. Did I mention I waited for Dr. Hurie? And waited and waited. I hate waiting.

"I see you are ready to go," he said, smiling, as he entered my room. I practically jumped out of the bed. I was so excited to get out of the hospital.

"Not that the service wasn't great, but I am ready to go home." I smiled back.

He loosened the gown and looked at his handiwork. "It looks good. I'll have the nurse come and take the IV out, and then you can go," he announced.

"Ah…what about the drains?" I asked, slightly confused.

"The drains will be kept in for about three to four weeks," he answered. "You will continue to empty each one three times a day and keep a log on the contents. Around the middle of the second week you will notice that there won't be as much fluid, and then you can empty them accordingly. That's all I heard. I could not get past the fact that I would have to keep the drains in for almost a month. Every once in a while I would catch another word, but I kept coming back to "drains for a month," "empty," and "keep log." I had assumed I was done with this whole situation. He continued, but I never heard, "I will refer you to oncology, and they will set up an appointment. Hopefully we can coordinate that appointment with the removal of the drains and the staples."

Removal of the drains…did I hear something about staples?

"I'll have my office call you in a week or so and set up the appointment."

Call office? No. They will call?

"The nurse will go over a set of instructions for you to follow before you can leave. Candace, you need to start exercising your right arm. I see that you are favoring it."

Of course I favor my right arm! It hurts!

"Do you have any questions?"

"No, I don't think so." I answered. Surely I had that dazed look again. It seemed it was becoming a habit, and I was getting tired of it. Of course I did not have any questions. Once again everything was going too fast. I honestly thought that this was a done deal. And now I find out I have to leave the drains in for a month or more and come back sometime. But I don't know when. I don't know if he said he was going to take the staples out first or the drains or was it the other way around?

"Candace, you are going to be fine. I'll see you in a month or so." Dr. Hurie patted my shoulder. "Have a safe trip home," he said as he left the room.

For the first time I could honestly say I was angry. I figured I had been through enough, and I really thought it was over. Dr. Hurie had removed the cancer, and I assumed he would remove the drains, and I would be able to go home, and it would be done. This was simply not acceptable. The demons were back. They were playing their evil little mind games. By the time Leon arrived I was in quite a state of mind, and he could tell I was not happy.

He looked at me. "You can't go home?" he asked. He knew something was up.

I wonder if his first clue was my pacing back and forth! I thought sarcastically.

"Oh, I get to go home, but I have to come back in a month or so because they are going to leave the drains in. And then he said something about the stitches, but I was so upset about the drains I didn't really catch what he said."

"Candace, it's okay. If we have to come back, we have to come back," Leon said calmly.

I glared at him. *Get a grip. So you have to go home with a couple of drains. So you have to come back in a month and have them removed. Why are you making a mountain out of a mole hill?* My anger subsided. He was right. *Lord, thank you for Leon. He is my shoulder to lean on.*

I took a deep breath. "I guess you're right. It's not a big deal. I was just hoping when I walked out of this hospital I would be done with the whole thing. But coming back in a month or so won't be so bad," I said as my mood was lifting.

"Are you ready then?" he asked.

"You betcha. Let's get out of here. It's time to go home." We gathered what few things I had brought and left the building. I was free, and it felt good. The demons were back in their place.

* * * * * * * * * * * * *

The cold front had moved out of the area, and it was a balmy ten degrees. I took a long, deep breath of the fresh, cold air. It stung my lungs, but it felt good to be outside. Leon had warmed the car so it was nice and toasty when we got in. It was time to go home.

The trip home was uneventful. The roads were clear of ice and snow. Leon and I made some small talk but we mostly listened to the radio. He told me that my mother was going to have dinner tonight so I didn't have to worry about cooking. I wasn't worried about cooking. In fact it was the last thing on my mind. But it was important to my mother, and if she wanted to cook that was okay with me. She was a great cook.

We arrived back into Glendive around 3:00 p.m. It was absolutely wonderful to be back in my home. I was pleasantly surprised at the number of get-well cards and flowers I had already received. I was humbled by the gestures. Kelly had left a note letting us know that dinner was at 5:00, and she and Chris would meet us over at my mom's. I walked around looking at everything as if it were the first time when Katie (the cat) came up from downstairs.

Katie had quite a strut! She held her head high and her tail stuck straight up. She marched right over to me and began to rub against my legs, meowing the entire time. I bent down to pet her, *BIG Mistake as the pain shot through my body*! I retreated to a chair. She jumped on my lap and proceeded to give me cat kisses letting me know that she missed me too. My heart filled with appreciation.

Then she firmly planted herself on my lap. Leon was busy unloading the car. I rested my head on the back of the chair and closed my eyes for a few minutes. Initially I had planned to go back to work on Wednesday but decided that I was going to take the rest of the week off and return to work on Monday, February 26. It was nice to be home, and I deserved to pamper myself a little. Plus I needed to start working on using my right arm a little more.

"Sorry, Katie, as nice as this is I have things to do," I said as I gently lifted her off. I could tell she was offended that her comfort was interrupted so soon. But not one to hold a grudge she jumped back on the chair and curled up where I had sat. I wasn't sure if she really missed me or my body heat!

I called work and talked with my supervisor, first to let her know I was home and secondly to get the okay to take more time off. I had plenty of sick-leave coming. I had only taken maybe a day or two a year since I had started working. Then I called my mother to let her know we were home and assured her that I was hungry. I had barely hung up the phone when it rang. Calls from my dad, brother and Leon's family followed one after another. And then friends began to call. Like I said earlier, news travels fast in a small town! I answered the same questions over and over again. I was getting to the point I didn't want to answer the phone anymore. I appreciated the concern but I was tired and sore and just wanted to relax. I couldn't wait for dinner.

Leon and I arrived at my mother's first. The aroma from the food simmering on the stove filled the house. It was wonderful. But my mom looked tired. I was sure certain it was from worry. She had already lost two brothers to cancer and I know she feared she might lose her daughter too. I was positive her demons were painting a pretty good picture in her mind too! I guess I would have felt the same way if my daughter had just been told she had cancer.

My mother and I were very close. Over the years our roles of mother and daughter had on occasion reversed. There were times when I had to take care of her, especially during her separation from my dad. So I wasn't surprised when my maternal instinct kicked in immediately. I had to protect her. I assured her everything was just fine as she gently hugged me. My mother would have done anything to make it better. Unfortunately there wasn't anything she could do— except cook! And let me tell you that was not a good thing...it was a great thing!

It wasn't long before Chris and Kelly showed up. I held each child close to me for long moment. Neither one pulled away from my embrace until I let go. It was hard to hold back the tears. Over dinner I retold my story, again. At the end I assured them that everything was going to be fine. *I seemed to be saying that a lot. I wonder if I was reassuring them or me.* But I could tell that everyone was still worried. It seemed that if I barely moved one of them would ask if I needed anything. It was something I was not used to and it was kind of nice. *I think I could get used to that kind of treatment!*

After recounting the last couple of days the conversation finally moved away from cancer to things in general. For a moment cancer was not the "hot" topic. The kids talked about how their week had gone. And then as we normally would do we began reminiscing about little things that happened in the past. When my mother lived in Coeur d'Alene, Idaho, the children went to visit her for a week. I think Chris was around ten years old and Kelly eight years old at the time. One day she took them to a water park for the day. After much persuading, Chris finally convinced my mother to go down the "big" slide with him. I couldn't imagine it because my mother was really afraid of water! Picture it...they come down the slide at a pretty good pace. They both land in the water. My mother is frantically trying to get her feet underneath her when Chris reaches for her as he is frantically trying to get his feet under him! In his panic he accidentally grabs her swimsuit and pulls the top down to her waist just as she was standing up. She is now standing in about two to three feet of water, totally exposed from the neck down—in front of God and everyone! She tried desperately to pull her top back up, but Chris was still hanging on for dear life! We laughed. It hurt so very much but it felt so very good to laugh. With every giggle, I could see the tension leave my mother and children's face. It felt good to be with my family.

Unfortunately all good things must come to end. As much as I was enjoying this time with my family, the pain was starting to wear on me. It was time to go home. I dreaded breaking the moment but I really needed to go home. As I struggled to get up the chair the worry returned to everyone's face. Cancer was back in the forefront. I hugged my mother and again reassured her that I was going to be just fine. She held me close almost like she was afraid to let go. I let her. When she released me there were tears in her eyes.

"I love ya, Ma!" I said with a big grin on my face. "Supper was fantastic. You are such a wonderful cook. Thanks." I hugged her again. "Sorry to eat and run. I'll call you tomorrow, okay?" I tried to act as if it had been any other time we had been over for a meal. She smiled back but said nothing. "Trust me, Mom. Everything is going to be just fine," I reassured her again.

We all left at the same time. "I need some pain medicine," I announced to Leon as we got in the car. It was the first time that I could honestly say I was in real pain. Between the emotional stress, driving in a car for almost four hours, sitting and visiting for more than three hours, it had been a long day.

I struggled to get out of the car. The pain was beginning to take over. I felt vulnerable and weak. I needed something to help relieve it, and I needed it now. I couldn't get into the house fast enough.

"Leon, could you get me a couple of pills, please?" I said as I made my way to the chair in the living room. I didn't have the strength to look for them at this point. I could tell by the look on my children's faces that they were worried. My mask of strength was disintegrating as the pain racked my body. I couldn't hide it. Leon returned with two pills and a glass of water. I took them quickly.

"I want to take one more." I stated. He was going to argue with me, but he could tell by the look in my eyes there was no point. He brought me one more. I took it. I laid my head back and closed my eyes. We all sat there waiting for the medication to do its stuff. No one said a word. The only sound was the ticking of the clock and soft breathing. What seemed to be an eternity but in reality was only fifteen minutes, the pain pills started to work. I could feel the pain lesson with every passing minute. I finally opened my eyes. I smiled affectionately at Leon, Chris, Kelly and Katie who were all waiting patiently for me to make the next move. I don't think they had ever seen me this vulnerable before.

"It's been quite a day," I said nonchalantly. "What time is it?"

"It's 8:35," Kelly answered. "Are the pills working?"

"Yes, I feel sooo much better," I answered. "What is your schedule tomorrow?" I asked hoping to change the subject and talk about something else. Katie moved from Kelly's lap and jumped into mine. She immediately curled up, planning to make a night of it. I gently petted her, and I could tell she was deeply appreciative by her loud purring.

Kelly answered my question, and Chris filled in with his schedule as well. Soon Leon, Kelly, and Chris were chatting about one thing and then another. I watched and listened to their exchange. Suddenly this enormous overwhelming feeling of gratefulness came over me. It was at that very moment I realized how truly fragile life was and how precious each moment I had with my family would become. It was the first time I understood the enormity of my diagnosis. I had cancer. I could die. I bowed my head and concentrated on petting Katie. I struggled to hold back the tears. Katie looked up at me as if she knew I was struggling and wanted to comfort me. I smiled and continued to pet her. I looked at my husband, my son, and my daughter, their voices and soft laughter filling the room. It was good to be home.

Thank you, God, for these wonderful gifts. I am so very blessed, I prayed silently and closed my eyes again.

⊶⟹ ⟸⊷

The best things are nearest: breath in your nostrils, light in your eyes, flowers at your feet, duties at your hand, the path of God just before you. Then do not grasp at the stars, but do life's plain, common work as it comes, certain that daily duties and daily bread are the sweetest things of life.

—Robert Louis Stevenson

Chapter Six
It Is Said, "Whatever Doesn't Kill You, Makes You Stronger"

The arctic front had finally moved out of the area. The weatherman forecasted much warmer temperatures. It was about time. The winter had been a long one. The sun was shining and it was a typical February morning with one exception. I didn't have to go to work and it was nice. I sent Leon, Chris and Kelly on their merry way out the door. I was sore but surprisingly feeling pretty good. I did pop two pain pills immediately. After last night I was determined to never let the pain get that bad again. Although I had taken more pain medication since I got home than I ever did in my entire stay in the hospital, I was no fool. I learned very quickly that I needed to stay on top of the pain.

I continued to favor my right arm. I knew that I had to start working with it or I was going to be in big trouble later on. But I figured I would deal with it later. I had big plans for the day and it did not include stretching or reaching with my right arm! First things first, I emptied each of the drains and logged its contents. I couldn't wait to get them out!

Next I did the best I could to tidy up the house. And then it was off to get caught up on my soaps. The only time I could watch them was when a holiday fell on a Monday or Friday. But I discovered you could go months without seeing one and still figure out the plot almost instantly. I grabbed a cup of coffee and settled into the couch. Katie was giddy because there was a warm lap she could snuggle into during the day. I grabbed the remote and channel surfed. I giggled. This was something that I rarely had the opportunity to do. I had the whole house to myself. We both settled in to what promised to be a good day.

Unfortunately it seemed that I had barely got comfortable when the phone rang. I struggled to get up. It was difficult to get out of the couch without straining. *Won't do that again,* I said to myself reaching for the receiver. "Hello," I said as I walked back to the couch, phone in tow.

"Hello, may I speak to Candace...eedee?" The person on the other end asked.

"It's pronounced i-dee." I answered back. "This is she."

"This is Dr. Twill's office. I am calling to schedule your appointment."

"Ah...who is Dr. Twill?" I asked slightly confused.

"Dr. Twill is an oncologist. I would like to schedule..." she started to say.

"Excuse me," I interrupted. "What is an oncologist?"

"It's a doctor that specializes in the cancer field," she answered back. "I would like to schedule an appointment with you to see Dr. Twill."

"Why do I have to see a cancer doctor?" I asked, getting more confused. "I just had surgery, and the cancer is gone." I felt stupid, and I hate that word.

"This was a referral made by Dr. Hurie. I am calling to set up an appointment to review your treatment plans."

"What treatment plans? I thought this was a done deal," I stated. Suddenly I had an ache in the pit of my stomach.

"Dr. Twill will go over the results of your tests and set up a treatment plan for chemotherapy. Will Tuesday the 27th at 10:00 a.m. work for you?"

I was stunned. *Chemotherapy? Are you serious? I honestly thought this whole ordeal was over! I have to have chemotherapy?*

"Candace, will the 27th work for you?" the person on the other end repeated.

"Ah, I guess so," I answered back sheepishly. *The demons began making their plans.* "Tuesday the 27th. What time did you say?

"Tuesday the 27th at 10:00 a.m. with Dr. Twill. The oncology department is located on the second floor of the clinic. Do you know where the clinic is?"

"Yes, I think I do. I'll find it." I stammered back. "Will I have to stay overnight?" I managed to ask.

"No, you shouldn't have to stay the night. Your appointment and protocol shouldn't last more than two hours," she said. "Okay, Candace, I have you down for Tuesday the 27th at 10:00 a.m. to see Dr. Twill."

"Okay," was all I could muster as I hung up the phone. I was shocked and confused. *The demons began their slow ascent. They were bringing their suitcases. They were planning to stay for a long time.*

I knew very little about chemotherapy. I remembered when one of my uncles had to have chemotherapy. He had lost all his hair, got very sick and lost lots of weight. Was the same thing going to happen to me? Why did I need chemotherapy? I really thought that once the breast was removed so was the cancer. I couldn't grasp the fact that I needed to have chemotherapy. Did that mean I still had cancer? I felt sick to my stomach. Anxiety and fear began their assault. This was a revolting turn of events.

I turned the TV off. There was no way I could sit, watch and enjoy something so far from reality. I was living in the now and it certainly had a lot more drama to it. I jumped when the phone rang.

"Hello," I said hesitantly because I wasn't sure I wanted to answer it. I did not want any more surprises or bad news.

"Good morning," my mom said. "How are you feeling?"

"Okay," I said as I tried to get control of myself. Again my instinct to protect my mother kicked in. "I am busy doing nothing. I am not used to that." We continued to talk about little things in general, like the weather finally turning into a tolerable cold, what her plans were for the day, what I was going to do the rest of the day and so on. All through our conversation the demons would sneak into my thoughts and I struggled to keep them at bay. We finally said our good-byes. I ended the conversation by reassuring her I was going to be just fine and no there wasn't anything I needed at the moment. I hung up the phone. Wow, this day was not turning out the way I had pictured it. Even the demons didn't know what to think. I couldn't believe I was going to have chemotherapy! I honestly thought that the surgery had taken care of everything.

I took a long, hard deep breath and gathered myself together. I called Leon and broke the news that we were headed back to Billings sooner that we had planned. He had lots of questions, which of course I couldn't answer. Then I called my work to let them know I wouldn't be back until the end of the following week. At this rate I wouldn't have many sick days left.

"Might as well start doing my arm exercises," I said out loud, feeling slightly sorry for myself. "This day is ruined anyway." Without much thought but with great determination I reached for the sky with my right arm. I was abruptly stopped when the tension and pain from my muscle refused to go further than a quarter of the way. I slowly brought my arm back down to my side. This was going to be much more difficult than I expected. This time I slowly raised my arm. I stretched it as far as the taut muscle would allow and held it there for a moment. It was very painful, but in a strange kind of way, it felt good. It kept the demons away, and I felt like I was doing something constructive instead of feeling sorry for myself. I repeated the procedure ten times. I made a mental note to repeat this at least twice a day.

Obviously this wasn't turning out at all the way I had planned it. Instead of enjoying my time off recuperating from something I thought was over, I would be spending time worrying about the "What ifs" for the rest of the week. The demons were busy making plans to make the rest of the day miserable. Why put myself through that?

"It's time to take control of this situation. I will not feel sorry for myself!" I said out loud. "I am going back to work. At least it will keep my mind busy most of the day."

With that challenge resolved I decided I would surprise everyone by making a big supper. I figured bad news is taken much better on a full stomach.

Leon got home first. I could tell he had a lot of questions. I asked him to wait until I broke the news to the kids at supper. Then we could collectively discuss the issue. He respectfully agreed.

Chris and Kelly were not very happy when I told them I had to have chemo. There were lots of questions and of course I had absolutely no answers. I also informed everyone that I was going back to work tomorrow. No one tried to persuade me not to go back. We spent the rest of the meal in quiet. There wasn't much more to be said I guess. After supper we cleaned up the kitchen and each of us went our own separate ways. We were all absorbed in our own thoughts. I could see worry on everyone's face. But at this point I didn't have the strength to reassure them that everything was going to be all right because the truth was I just didn't know. I honestly thought that once the surgery was over, the whole ordeal was over. I really believed that the cancer was gone and I could get on with my life. But things don't always go the way we plan.

It was a long evening but finally 10:00 rolled around. I slowly readied myself for bed. I emptied the drains and logged the contents. I couldn't wait to get them out. I looked over the incision to make sure there wasn't any indication of an infection. Everything thing looked okay. I put my pajamas on with care. I continued to favor my right arm. Finally I made my way downstairs to say good night. I was almost to the end of the last step when the pain shot through me again. It took my breath away. I stopped. Leon looked up to see what I was doing.

"Are you all right?" he asked as he hurried over to where I was standing.

I just nodded, breathing very slowly. He stood beside me. He didn't know what to do. Again as quickly as it came it went away. "I just had a little pain by one of the drains." I told him, exhaling deeply. "I don't know what's up, but I can't wait to get these drains out. I think I will call Dr. Hurie's office to see if this normal."

"Candace if you have another pain, I think you should see if you can get an appointment to see him while we are in Billings," Leon said, concern written all over his face.

I smiled at him. "I will be fine," I said as I patted him on the arm. "I just came down to say good night."

"Are you sure you're okay? he asked as I made my way to the kid's room and said my good nights.

"I think I'm just tired. It's been quite a day," I said as I leaned over to give him a kiss. "Good night, hon; love you."

"Good night. Love you," he returned. "I will be up after the news." I nodded and carefully headed back up the stairs. I was uneasy about the pain attacking me again. It was awful. Thankfully I made it up without incident.

I made my way to the bedroom, turned down the bed and climbed in. I said my prayers. I always feel revived after prayer because I believe in the power of prayer. But unfortunately tonight I said my prayer without conviction. I was weak and letting the demons take over. They were gathering strength by feeding on my fear and pain. I didn't know how to stop them. It was a long and restless night.

* * * * * * * * * * * *

I surprised everyone at work by showing up the next morning. There were lots of questions. The number-one question was, "Why are you favoring your right arm?" I answered them all the best I could. I was grateful that no one tried to avoid me. I appreciated that.

I spent the rest of the week getting caught up from the days I missed and planning for what I was going to do in the next couple of months. On Friday the staff hosted a pot-luck welcome-back luncheon. There were still some questions, and again I answered them the best I could. I said nothing about the chemo. I had no information about it, so why bother bringing it up at this point?

As was the usual case at these functions someone would start reminiscing about one thing or another, and the laughter would begin. I got caught up in the moment and told them about the time my supervisor and I went to Circle for a meeting. Circle is a small town about 40 miles northwest of Glendive. I drove. It was the middle of January and there was snow and ice on the roads.

I was new to the position, and my supervisor was going with me to introduce me to the group. The group consisted of County Commissioners, the Mayor, and about five other distinguished people in the community. Our meeting was at the Senior Center which is located on Main Street next to the grocery store. My intention was to impress everyone so I dressed accordingly. I wore a business suit (with a skirt) and high heels. Picture it: I proceeded to get out of the car when my shoe slips on the ice and my left foot slides under the car. The rapid sideways motion caused my body to jolt severely to the left causing my right leg to spring up and get lodged between the steering wheel and dashboard. Thank goodness the heat from my hands had helped them stick to the ice which had stopped me from totaling falling out of the car and landing on my face.

I heard Laura whisper, "Oh my God!" as she frantically got out of the car to try to help me. Unfortunately she didn't know how!

Finally after a few unsuccessful attempts, I managed to gently lay myself down on the pavement. I would like to say gracefully, but I can't! I looked up from where I was lying on the ice and snow, and a man is standing motionless, wide-eyed, mouth open, and with a bag of groceries in each arm. He was stunned by the commotion! At last I got my feet under me, stood up, and brushed the snow off my suit.

The man finally overcame his astonishment and asked, "Are you hurt?"

I managed to say, "Only my pride."

Everyone laughed. It felt so good to laugh. I laughed so hard it hurt. And it hurt so bad that I had to take the rest of the day off. But it was a good way to end the week.

* * * * * * * * * * * * * *

Leon and I left for Billings around 6:00 a.m. Tuesday morning. It was still dark outside. The nurse said it shouldn't take more than two hours. We planned on making it a one-day trip so we didn't pack anything for overnight. We did, however bring an empty ice cream bucket and wash cloth...just in case I got sick. I was not looking forward to this visit.

"So, what do you think will happen?" I asked Leon.

"Happen with what?" he asked.

"The chemotherapy," I answered back. We hadn't talked about it much since I had announced to everyone that I had to have chemotherapy. My mother had gotten visibly upset when I told her. The children didn't know what to think. Leon didn't know what to say. The end result no one really talked about. Now that Leon and I were in the car again with 3½ hours on our hands I thought it would be a good time to talk about it.

"You know about as much as I do," he replied.

"This is what I think. If I have to have chemo once a month for six months, that will mean they got all the cancer, and the chemo is just a precautionary measure. If I have to have chemo twice a month for six months, then it's a little more serious than I thought. If I have to have chemo once a week for six months...well, that probably means I am in big trouble." I looked at him and said, "Let's pray I only have to have chemo once a month for six months."

"Let's pray," he said. We sat quietly for a moment.

"There is one other thing." I said after I said my prayer. "I need you to come into the exam room with me. I think I need another set of ears to hear everything they are telling me. I seem to be missing or not understanding a lot of information they are giving me. I am getting tired of these surprises."

"No problem," he answered.

"And, do you remember before surgery I asked you what if I had cancer and the doctor told me I was dying? You didn't say anything, and I didn't push the subject. But now I know I have cancer. I need to know if I am going to die. Leon, I want you to ask the doctor if I am dying."

He kept his eyes on the road. Finally he said, "Yes, I will ask the doctor if you are dying."

"Thank you." We spent the rest of the trip in quiet. I spent most of my time silently talking to God.

We had no trouble finding the clinic and we arrived early as usual. Butterflies flitted around in my stomach as we walked into the clinic. I was scared, plain and simple. We climbed the one flight of stairs to the second floor. We followed the signs that pointed to oncology. My heart fell when we walked in. There were three patients already seated waiting their turn. One was woman with a scarf on her head. She must have lost her hair. There was a man reading a magazine. And then…there was a little girl no more than seven or eight years old. She looked up from the puzzle she was trying to put together. Her eyes were clear and blue. She smiled. I noticed immediately that she had no hair. Tears filled my eyes and I had to look away. She stopped what she was doing and bounded over to her dad and crawled into his lap and gave him a hug. He hung onto her until she let go. He looked tired.

"Hi, little one," the nurse said as she approached the two of them. "How are you doing today?" She reached out her hand, and the little girl grabbed it.

"I am doing great," the little girl replied. "Except I get so tired sometimes. Dad says I play too hard and I…" was all I could hear her say as she exited the room with the nurse. Her dad went back to his magazine. It was obvious they had done this before.

I felt so guilty about how sorry I was feeling for myself. I could not imagine nor do I ever want to feel what that parent was going through. I felt awful. Reality gave me a cold slap in the face. I deserved it.

I checked in with the receptionist and again with the paperwork. I put it into perspective and completed as I was asked. It didn't take long and I was called back. Leon came with me.

"How are you today?" the nurse asked.

"I don't know." I answered.

She smiled and she opened the examination room. "Dr. Twill will be with you in a moment," she said.

"I sometimes think this is the worst part…waiting for the doctor." I said making small talk. We just sat there occasionally looking at each other.

The door opened, and Dr. Twill entered. He was around six feet four, and he stood straight as an arrow, making him look taller. He reached his hand out as he introduced himself. "Good morning. I am Dr. Twill. You must be Candace," he said as he shook my hand then released it and reached for Leon. "And you are…" he asked.

"Leon, I am Candace's husband."

"Good morning, Leon," he said. He sat down at the desk. He casually thumbed through my file. "I see that the results from the biopsy came back positive. Probably why you are here," he said with a smile. "Are you ready for the next step?"

"I don't know. I don't know what the next step is," I answered nervously.

"The next step is chemotherapy. I will start you on the Cooper regimen for stage II breast carcinoma," he said as he continued to review my file. "Let's see how many lymph nodes were involved?" He tried to hide his surprise when he said, "Oh, fifteen out of fifteen!" He went back to my chart. Leon and I sat there quietly waiting for him to continue. Leon glanced at me. I mouthed, "Ask him," and tilted my head towards the doctor.

"Dr. Twill, is Candace going to die?" Leon asked tentatively.

Dr. Twill looked up for the chart. "Not if I can help it," he simply stated. "I have to admit that I am surprised by the lymph involvement. I want to call the Mayo Clinic to see if I need to add anything to the protocol. We work closely with the Mayo Clinic, especially in advanced stages. I will be right back," he said as he left the room.

"I guess that's good news," I said, not sure if I was relieved or not. "I hope I don't need to take it more than once a month for 6 months."

It wasn't long before Dr. Twill returned. "The Clinic confirmed the treatment. I thought maybe I would have to add something, but it was agreed the Cooper regimen is appropriate. Okay, let's go over the protocol. You will orally take 60 mg. cytoxan daily. There are three drugs that you will be given intravenously; fluorouracil or 5FU, methotrexate, and vincristine. I am also starting you on prednisolone. You will take that orally for 70 days. You will start with 30 mg and decrease gradually to 2.5 mg. The nurse will go over the side effects of each drug as she administers them today."

"How often do I have to have chemotherapy?" I asked, bravely.

"You will take the cytoxan daily and the injections once a week for one year."

I thought I was going to fall off the chair! *Excuse me! Did I hear him right? My worst nightmare had just come true! I was going to be on chemotherapy for one year! No! Someone please tell me I heard him wrong!*

"Excuse me. Did you say I had to take this once a week for one year?" I asked in disbelief.

"Yes," he said. "Because of the massive lymph node involvement it is imperative that you undergo an aggressive treatment plan." He paused, looking for a way to describe it to me so I would understand. "Because all of your lymph nodes showed cancer there is a good chance there are cells floating around in your body. It's important to try to get to them before they attach to something, which most likely would be your bones. You will have to let me know if you ever feel achy."

You could have knocked me over with a feather. I looked at Leon. He was pale. We were both in a state of shock.

"Brenda will be here in a few minutes to start your protocol. Occasionally after surgery some swelling, called lymphedema, can occur on the arm on the side of the surgery. To prevent swelling it is recommended that you do not have blood drawn or injections in that arm. It is also recommended that have your blood pressure taken on your left side." He paused and looked at me. "I will need to see you once a month for the first year, then once every three months for one year, once every six months for the next two years, and then once a year after that. Before each visit I would like you to have your blood work and x-rays done. Brenda will set up an appointment for the following weeks." He rose to leave. "Candace, I am going to do my very best to help you through this." With that said, he left the room.

I looked at Leon. He had a dazed look, too. We just sat there. We didn't know what to do.

"Well," I started to say when the door opened.

"Hi, Candace, my name is Brenda. Please come with me, and we can begin your protocol," she said as she led us to another room. There were five recliners. Each chair was divided from the others by a curtain. She told me to sit down. I obeyed.

"Leon, you can wait for Candace in the waiting room. It should only take about thirty minutes," she said as she pointed to the exit. Leon obeyed. We were very good at following orders.

"Make yourself comfortable while I get ready," she said as she left. I picked the chair closest to me and sat down. I was not comfortable. I didn't know what to expect, and I was very nervous. Then I remembered that little girl. *I wonder which chair she sat in,* I thought. Again a surge of guilt passed through me. *There are definitely worse things, Candace,* I thought harshly to myself. *Get over yourself!* I bowed my head and silently prayed for forgiveness for not trusting in Him, and I asked that He continue to give that little girl and her family the strength and courage to face her challenge.

Brenda returned with a tray. "I will go over each injection as I give it to you. I will also send a sheet home that has more in-depth information," she said as she prepared the area. "I encourage you to read it thoroughly. You can call us anytime if you have questions." She sat down on a little stool next to me. "Which side did you have your surgery on?" she asked.

"My right side."

"I will need your left arm then," she said as she took my left arm and wrapped a strap around it. She tapped my arm looking for a vein. "Did Dr. Twill explain to you to not have blood drawn or injections in your right arm?"

"Yes, he told me about the possibility of swelling." I was amazed I had heard what he said. I seemed to miss a lot of the conversations lately. "Is that a forever thing?" I asked.

"Generally lymphedema can show up as much as a year later. You have great veins," she said as she slipped the needle into my vein and hooked me up to an IV machine. I was glad she was happy about my great veins. "The purpose of the IV drip is to help the drugs get into your system faster," she informed me. "Okay. Are you ready?"

"As ready as I'll ever be," I smiled at her.

"This first injection is fluorouracil or commonly referred to as 5-FU," she said as she slowly inserted the needed into the intravenous port. "Side effects may include, and I stress the word, *may,* because not everyone experiences all the side effects; I want you to know that…" she was looking for a sign that I was hearing what she was saying. "Side effects *may* include sores in your mouth, easy bruising or bleeding, bloody or tarry stools, fever or chills, vomiting, or hand-foot syndrome, which causes a tingling sensation, pain, swelling, or tenderness of the hands and feet. Five-FU can lower your immune activity, making you susceptible to infections, so try to avoid contact with people who have a cold, flu, or other contagious infections."

I looked at her incredulously. "Are you serious?" I thought as I watched her place the empty needle in the disposal. This didn't sound good at all.

"This next injection is called methotrexate. Common side effects may include chills and fever; hair loss; infertility or irregular periods; loss of appetite; sensitivity to sunlight, so avoid the sun, sunlamps, or tanning booths; unusual tiredness; vomiting, and lowered resistance to infection." She looked at me. I was sure she was trying to see if I understood anything that she said.

"You mentioned hair loss. Am I going to lose my hair?" I finally managed to ask. I was sick to my stomach, and I was sure it wasn't from the medicine, at least not yet. I don't consider myself vain in any way, but for some reason the thought of me losing my hair made me ill.

"Again, these are possible side effects, and yes, you may lose your hair," she said, trying to reassure me. "If you do lose your hair, you won't notice it for a month or so. You may only see some thinning." She rose to dispose of the needle. I couldn't believe what I was hearing. I've heard the saying, "What doesn't kill you will make you stronger." I do believe I was going to test that theory to see if it was really true!

"Last but not least is vincristine," she said lightly, trying to soften the mood. "Common side effects include constipation, hair loss, nausea or vomiting. You may experience some dizziness or lightheadedness, so be aware, and do not drive if you notice it. Other side effects may include vision changes, numbness or tingling of your fingers and toes, mouth sores, or unusual bruising or bleeding. Also, empty your bladder frequently. When you feel you have to go to the bathroom, go," she said as she removed the needle from the port. "Do you have any questions?"

I am sure that I had a blank look on my face, because I was dumbfounded by the information she had just shared with me. I had to do this once a week for one year—that's fifty-two times. No, make that fifty-one times! Words like "hair loss," "vomiting," "sore mouth," "tingling something or other" kept replaying in my mind. I felt like this was all a bad dream. I didn't have the clear-headedness to ask any questions.

"Dr. Twill has also given you written prescriptions for cytoxan and prednisolone," she continued when I didn't answer her. "Common side effects that may occur with cytoxan are appetite loss, infertility, hair loss, general unwell feeling, skin rash, vomiting, and weakness."

There were those words again..."hair loss," "weakness," "appetite loss."

"Prednisolone may cause some dizziness; you may see an increase in your appetite, facial flushing, and unusual weight gain."

Excuse me; how can you lose your appetite, vomit, increase your appetite, and have unusual weight gain all at the same time? This was more than I could absorb.

"You can fill the prescriptions here at the clinic or at your pharmacy," she said as she handed me the prescriptions. She looked up at the IV drip. It was down to the last drop. "Okay, that should do it." She gently but quickly removed the needle from my arm. She applied pressure to the puncture and then covered it with a bandage. "How are you feeling?"

"I don't know," I answered as I struggled to get out of the chair. "I think it's too soon to tell."

"Stop by the desk and make an appointment for next week," she said as she ushered me to the waiting room. "If you have questions at any time, don't hesitate to call."

It was done. My first chemotherapy session was over. I looked for Leon. He looked up from the magazine that he was not really reading. He stood and walked over to me. I could see the questions in his eyes.

"I have to make an appointment for next week," I said before he could get a word in.

It was quick and painless. "My next appointment is next Tuesday, March 6, at 10:00 a.m. We are free to go." I could hardly wait to get out of there.

We walked to the car without saying a word. I was replaying the last thirty minutes in my head. It seemed so surreal. It was like I was having an out of body experience. The player I was watching looked like me, but it didn't seem real.

As we got into the car Leon finally asked, "How are you doing?"

"I'm okay," I said as he started the car. I looked at my watch. It was 11:15. "Are you hungry?" I asked.

"I hadn't thought about it," he answered.

"I am. Let's go eat."

"Seriously? he asked, surprised. "Where do you want to go?"

"Let's go to Perkins. The food there isn't too bad. We should beat the lunch-hour rush if we go now. And I think there is a pharmacy next door. I have two prescriptions I need to fill," I said as if I had not spent the last hour with a cancer doctor and had not just undergone chemotherapy. The truth was I was numb, but I was feeling okay. And I was hungry.

Leon looked at me.

"I know you have lots of questions," I said as he pulled out of the clinic parking lot. "Can we eat first? Then I will fill you in as to what is going to happen." We drove in silence to the restaurant. I was right. There was a pharmacy next to the restaurant. We left the prescriptions and went over to eat.

The waitress took our order. I mentioned how nice the weather had gotten and other trivial items. Leon gave a response when appropriate. Our lunch came. We both stared at our plates for a brief minute.

"I don't think I can eat," Leon announced as he continued to stare at the plate in front of him.

I looked at him and smiled. "I'm starved," I said as I took a bite, "and from what I've been told I am going to enjoy this meal." I said with my mouth full. I chewed and swallowed. "It could be the last one that will stay with me for a while," I said, trying to be a little funny. From the look on his face I didn't succeed.

"I don't think that is funny," he said as he sat back from the table.

""Hon, we are going to get through this. Everything will be okay. Please eat your lunch."

He looked at me. He took a deep breath and finally took a bite of his food. I ate a few more bites, and suddenly I wasn't hungry anymore, either. Again, both of us looked at the food on our plates. It was the first time we had ever left food on a plate.

"Let's go," I said. Leon asked the waitress for the bill, and we left. We picked up the two prescriptions. It was time to go home.

On our way I filled him in on what information I could actually remember. I told him about the possible hair loss. But I didn't tell him how that bothered me. I told him about the possibility of my getting sick and tired. I laughed. It was the first time "sick and tired" really had meaning. It was all I could remember. I opened the prescription package to refresh my memory about the possible side effects of the two medicines. I did remember that most of them had the same side effects. I read the list from the information sheet attached to the medication. Leon never said a word.

"Oh, this is interesting," I said as I was finishing the list. "One of the side effects of prednisolone is, "false sense of well-being." I think that is one side effect I will appreciate." I smiled. We had only traveled for about fifty miles when I felt the urge to go to the bathroom. Usually I could last at least until Forsyth, which is about one hundred miles east of Billings. But I remembered Brenda telling me not to hold it when I had to go.

"If there is an opportunity to turn off, I will need to use a restroom. I was told not to hold it. One of the side effects, you know."

Leon glanced over at me. "There is a turn-off about twenty miles down the road. Can you hold it that long?" he asked with genuine concern.

"Yes, I can hold it that long. I don't think one dose is going to do that much damage yet."

Leon stepped on the gas. Thank goodness the roads were clear of ice and snow. I fought back the tears. I wasn't surprised but I was overwhelmed by his concern. The poor guy had a long road ahead of him.

We spent the remainder of the trip home planning for the rest of the year. The first thing we needed to address was driving back and forth to Billings for my treatment. There had to be a way to have my chemo in Glendive. Driving 440 miles a week was just not acceptable. Next week I would talk with Dr. Twill and hopefully make different arrangements.

Our next discussion involved whether I would continue working or not. I wanted to work. I couldn't imagine sitting home all day with nothing but time on my hands. I knew the demons would take over! I reiterated that I *may* have these side effects, but until then it was important to keep things as normal as possible. We tried to cover all the bases, but the problem was we did not know how I was going to react to the chemo later on. I was hoping I wouldn't have any of those awful side effects.

And then suddenly, without warning, the sharp pain shot through me body! I gasped. Leon glanced over to see what the problem was. I tried to sit up as straight as I could. The pain was centered around the stitch on the lower drain. I took a deep breath and held it. Finally it passed. I relaxed.

"Wow, that was interesting." I managed to say. "This time it felt like a nerve was rudely awakened somewhere around the stitch on the lower tube! I cannot wait until I get these drains out. They are a real pain…literally!" I said, forcing a smile.

Leon had that worried look again. I didn't know what to say to him. I was worried too. I have to admit that really, really hurt. It seemed every time I had a pain it was getting worse. I have a high threshold for pain but that one took me for a loop. I hoped that it would not happen again. The rest of the trip Leon kept a cautious eye on me.

* * * * * * * * * *

Once again it felt good to be home. I was already tired from driving back and forth to Billings. The excitement of going to a "big city" had worn off. We definitely needed to solve this issue.

When I got into the house I decided the first thing I needed to do was empty my drains. I wasn't sure if that was going to make a difference, but I wasn't going to take any chances. I didn't want to feel that pain again ever! I finished cleaning the end of the tubes when I caught a glimpse of myself in the mirror. I realized I never took a really good look at myself. I've looked at the incision, but I never took a good look at my body. The brown gunk had been washed away. I gently touched the incision. There was still some redness and tenderness around the stitches. I felt a sadness wash over me. My right breast was gone, and it wasn't a pretty sight. I didn't like what I was seeing at all. I knew that unless I had reconstruction that this is how I would look forever. Could I live with that realization? I had eliminated reconstruction as an option. I did not want it. But did I want to look like this for the rest of my life? And then I realized I never asked Leon how he felt about having a wife with one breast. I know before the surgery he said it didn't matter to him but now that it was really gone does he feel the same way?

"Get a hold of yourself," I said out loud to the image in the mirror. "You are just tired at the moment." I put my shirt back on. "Anyway it is just a boob," I reminded myself. "Remember, it has no value." I hope I believed that soon!

It had been a long day. Although we were gone less than ten hours it seemed much, much longer. I was glad this day was over.

I announced my intentions to go to bed. I said my goodnights and "love you" to Leon, Chris, and Kelly. I wasn't sure if the chemo had started to work its magic, but I was totally exhausted.

I undressed and got into bed. I lay there, quietly replaying the events of the day over and over again. I closed my eyes. The demons immediately started to party. They were overzealous with joy. And their antics were mean and evil.

I could tell it was going to be a very, very long night again. And it was going to be a struggle to find something to be grateful for. It is hard to be grateful when you are feeling sorry for yourself. I would have to dig deep! But I was determined not to let the demons get the upper hand. I reminded myself the power of prayer. I reminded myself of God's never-ending love. I prayed with complete certainty in my belief that God is with me always! For the first time in a long time I feel asleep feeling strong.

It is not only blessed to give thanks; it is also of vital importance to our prayer in general. If we have noted the Lord's answers to our prayers and thanked Him for what we have received of Him, then it becomes easier for us, and we get more courage to pray for more.

—O. Hallesby

Chapter Seven
Acceptance Isn't Resignation

I woke up the next morning feeling better than I had for a long time. I had my first chemo protocol and survived it still intact. I felt like I could do this. *It is time to quit feeling sorry for myself and get on with living.* With renewed hope I headed for the kitchen to make breakfast. And then without any warning the pain struck again. I stopped in my tracks forcing myself to relax as it tormented my body and fear took over. Tears came to my eyes. And as suddenly as it appeared it went away. I knew something was not right, this was not normal. I slowly took a step forward and everything seemed fine. I shook off the demons and focused on making breakfast although I was worried the pain would return again. I didn't know what caused it and it was getting more and more frequent. I just knew it was one of the worst pains I had ever been through. I was definitely going to call Dr. Hurie for an appointment next Tuesday. I was not going to procrastinate this time.

* * * * * * * * * * * * *

We traveled back to Billings the following week for my second chemo treatment and to see Dr. Hurie. The pain was becoming more and more frequent. There was never any forewarning. It was always unexpected and it always took my breath away. I tried to hide it but when it hit it took control. I was devastated by the worry I could see in my family's eyes but there wasn't anything I could do about it. When it attacked it would almost take me to my knees. I had to stop whatever I was doing and wait until it was over. It was awful. The good news is it only lasted for about ten to fifteen seconds but it seemed forever and I always felt vulnerable afterwards. I couldn't wait to get the drains out.

My appointment with Dr. Hurie was at 8:00 a.m. so Leon and I went up the night before. We stayed at the same motel but this time we ate in because I never knew when I would have an attack. Morning could not come early enough.

We retired early and watched TV in bed. I found it difficult to get comfortable because it seemed no matter how I laid it would hurt. And the worst of it was it was getting to the point any kind of movement would trigger it. Did I mention I couldn't wait to get the drains out?

We watched TV until the news was over...or should I say Leon watched TV until the news was over. I spent most of the time trying to find a position that wouldn't trigger the pain. Finally I found lying in a fetal position seemed to work the best and I was able to relax, at least for a moment. Sleep eluded me. I was becoming emotionally fragile. I didn't know what was causing this intolerable pain. I think deep down I was afraid cancer was invading my body and I was dying. *The demons were winning their battle to control my thoughts.*

I could by tell Leon's soft breathing he had fallen asleep. I lay quietly afraid to move. Finally I managed to doze off when—bam, the pain racked my body. And this time it wasn't going away. I slowly got out of bed. I didn't want to wake Leon. I made my way to the bathroom, closed the door and fumbled for the light switch. At last the pain subsided. I took a deep breath and slowly exhaled. It was such a relief when the pain was gone and then—bam, it hit again.

I leaned against the wall taking slow, shallow breaths. I was beginning to think breathing was causing the pain. It was so intense I couldn't take it anymore. *The demons had won. They had me convinced I was dying.* Tears came to my eyes. I tried to hold them back but it was no use. I began to cry...no I began to bawl. I grabbed a towel to smother the sobs that were spewing uncontrollably from my mouth. I did not want Leon to hear me. The pain continued to attack my body as the flood gate of tears had been released. I couldn't stop. I thought neither would ever end. And then, what seemed to be an eternity both finally stopped. I continued to lean against the wall afraid to move. I was totally emotionally and physically exhausted. I finally understood what my mother meant.

She would say, "Someday you will be in pain, and you won't be able to think clearly, either. All you will be able to do is focus on the pain." My mother had been diagnosed with osteoarthritis years ago. There were days that she would be in so much pain she couldn't think straight, and I worried she was getting Alzheimer's. But she was right. When the pain hit I couldn't concentrate on anything else. It consumed me.

"Okay, God, we gotta talk. I know You don't give out more than a person can handle, but this is big one," I whispered as I started to pray. I closed my eyes and immediately the image of the little girl at the doctor's office popped into my head. I resented the image. I wanted to feel sorry for myself, but when I thought about children going through cancer it would put what I was going through into perspective. I couldn't feel sorry for myself, and I really wanted to feel sorry for myself.

"Dear God, I know you must be tired of me asking for the same things over and over again…but God, I do pray for your forgiveness. I pray for courage to deal with this awful disease and strength to fight my sin. And God, I pray I can abide by and accept your will as you guide me through these trying times. I know that you are with me, always." I took a long hard deep breath, and from the very depth of my soul I continued to pray. "I give it all to you, Lord. I give it all to you. You are my salvation, and I love you." I remained very still, and soon I began to feel better. I am always amazed and never surprised at the power of prayer. The demons had left. They knew they could never triumph over the power of prayer.

I slowly made my way back to bed. Again, bam—a pain hit me. I stood motionless until it passed. There were no more tears. I didn't feel sorry for myself anymore. I was in control again, and it felt good. But I admit it was a long, long night.

* * * * * * * * * * * *

Leon woke up around 5:30 to find me sitting in a chair. He immediately had that worried look on his face. I assured him I found I had less pain sitting up than lying down.

"When did you get up?" he asked.

"I moved to the chair shortly after midnight."

"Long night?" he asked.

"I've had better," I answered.

"Are you hungry?" he asked.

"No, I think I'll wait until the doctors' appointments are over, but you can eat something if you want. I would take a cup of coffee, though," I said smiling sweetly.

"I'll get dressed and get some coffee and the paper. Are you sure you're okay?" he asked.

"I am fine. I just want to..." I began when a pain shot through my body. Leon waited as I closed my eyes, lowered my head, and waited for it to pass, "...find out what is causing this pain." I continued to say. I looked at him and smiled. "See how quickly it comes and goes?"

"I'll get some coffee," he said as he finished dressing. "You okay?"

"Just thirsty!" I quipped. I was worried his frown would become permanent.

"I'm on my way," he said as he left the room.

He returned shortly with two hot cups of coffee and a newspaper. We had about two hours before my appointment with Dr. Hurie. Leon showered and got ready. I decided just to get dressed and shower when I got home. We spent the rest of the time sharing the paper and watching CNN on TV. The pain continued to hit off and on and it always took my breath away but it seemed I could handle it now.

The walk to the clinic was maybe, at the most five minutes. It was just across the street from the motel. My appointment with Dr. Hurie was at 8:00 a.m. True to form, I wanted to leave at 7:30. I am always early, it is such a habit. This morning I was hoping if I got there early, I would get in early and hopefully get these drains out sooner and since Leon and I had gotten up early we were ready to go.

We began the trek across the street at 7:30. We stepped off the curb when a pain shot through me. I grabbed for Leon's arm and we stopped in our tracks. I closed my eyes and breathed slowly waiting for it to pass and it did. We took another step and again, it hit me. We stopped and waited. It passed.

"Good thing we started early." I looked at Leon and smiled. The frown was buried deep in his forehead. "At this rate we will barely make it in time." He never said a word.

We took another step, and bam, it hit me again. We stopped and waited. This one seemed to last a little longer, but it finally subsided. By now we are in the middle of the street, and of course a car is heading towards us so we tried to pick up the pace, and bam, the pain hit hard again. I tried to take another step, but I had to stop. I couldn't move when I was in pain. The car stopped and waited, and finally the pain subsided. We took a couple more steps, and again it attacked me. Leon looked at the driver and shrugged. I wanted to get out of the way, but I could not move. Again the pain went away. We took a couple more steps, and again it hit hard. Thank goodness we were at least far enough so the car could go around us.

"Do you need help?" the driver asked as he pulled beside us.

"No, but thanks for asking." Leon responded. "It is just going to take us a while to get across the street."

I just smiled. And it did. It took us thirty minutes to get from the motel to the doctor's office. See? It pays to leave early!

Leon left me standing by the sitting area while he checked me in. The nurse looked at me. I was in the middle of a pain attack. She immediately called me back. With her help we slowly made our way back to the examining room. She graciously helped me get into the gown. I was grateful Dr. Hurie came in right away.

"I see you are having problems," he said as he looked over my chart. "Where is the pain located?"

"Around here," I said as I pointed to the lower drain. The movement triggered another attack.

"Let me help you to the table," he said as he gently guided me to the table. "I want to see what is causing this problem." I carefully sat on the end of the table.

"Can you lie back?" he asked.

"I can try," I said as I slowly lay down on the table. Another pain shot through me.

Dr. Hurie waited until the pain had gone. He had concern on his face, too. He cautiously opened the gown. He examined the area around the drains.

"I don't see anything unusual, but I am going to remove this drain and see if it relieves the problem." He grabbed a scissors and snipped the stitches that held the drain in place. He slowly pulled the tube through the hole in my skin, and whoosh…liquid spurted from the opening just as he finished pulling the drain out.

"This has never happened before!" he said with surprise as he reached for some paper towels to wipe off his jacket where the liquid had hit him. In fact there was fluid on the table and the floor as well! "The drain was plugged. No wonder you were in so much pain!" he said in amazement.

I sat up. I couldn't believe it. The pain was gone. It felt like the weight of the world had been lifted from my shoulders. I grinned from ear to ear. I felt like a new person!

"I am so sorry this happened to you," he said with genuine concern. "I have never had this happen before, and I am not sure how or why it happened."

"I am so happy the pain is gone," I said. It was such a relief!

"I think I am going to take the other drain out as well," he announced. I was overjoyed.

"The problem is the area will continue to fill with fluid for a while. You will have to have it aspirated probably once a week for the next four to six weeks."

"I am okay with that." I agreed wholeheartedly but didn't understand a thing he said. All I knew was that I wanted those drains out. I would do whatever I had to do as long as those drains were gone.

He skillfully removed the other drain. "How does that feel?" he asked as he examined the area.

"I cannot begin to tell you how good it feels not to be in pain," I said.

"Well, everything looks good. Remember you will have to be aspirated for a while. But it is healing nicely. I am still unsure as to why this happened," he said as he sat at the desk and wrote down a few notes.

He looked up and smiled. "I don't see any reason why I should have to see you again," he said. "Do you have any questions?"

"No, I don't think so."

He stood to leave. "Candace, you are going to get through this just fine," he said as he reached for my hand and shook it gently. "I wish you well." And then he left the room.

It was the last time I saw Dr. Hurie. He was a conscientious doctor who cared for his patients. And as much as I liked him, I was glad I could close this chapter. It felt so good to be pain free…well at least for the moment.

* * * * * * * * * * * * *

I walked into the waiting room, my head held high, ready to take on chemo. Leon looked up, totally surprised by the transformation. I smiled.

"What happened?" he asked.

"Dr. Hurie removed the drains. I guess one of them plugged and was causing the pain and pressure. The pain is gone."

"Thank goodness," he said, sighing deeply.

"Now let's get this chemo stuff out of the way and go home," I said with a new attitude. I felt as though I could take on the world and win.

The oncology department was just down the hall from Dr. Hurie's office. It was only 9:15 and my appointment wasn't until 10:00. Imagine that…we were early! I regretted not getting a little something to eat before I had seen Dr. Hurie, because for the first time in a long time I was hungry. I decided there wasn't enough time to grab something before my appointment with chemo and figured I wouldn't be hungry after the treatment. Now that the pain was gone I had returned to my optimistic self and decided that since I wanted to lose a little weight this was the perfect opportunity. I settled for a hot cup of coffee after I checked in with the receptionist.

Leon and I waited patiently. There were two other patients waiting also. I kept wondering if the little girl would show up. I was hoping she wouldn't. It broke my heart every time I visualized her. Finally the nurse called me back. My first appointment was with Dr. Twill to discuss having my treatments in Glendive. The meeting was short and sweet. Dr. Twill agreed that I could have my weekly chemo treatments in Glendive. He would make the arrangements with Dr. Shorn, and I was elated. He also made arrangements to see me either in Sidney or Miles City. Sidney was only fifty miles north of Glendive and Miles City was seventy-five miles west of Glendive. This was working out better than I had hoped.

I had my second chemotherapy treatment without incident. Afterwards I felt fine. *This is going to be a piece of cake,* I thought, arrogantly. *Two down, and fifty to go...no problem!*

"Let's go home," I said to Leon as I returned to the waiting room.

"What did Dr. Twill say about having your chemo in Glendive?" Leon asked. I filled him in with all the details. It was a relief for both of us.

"Are you hungry?" I asked as we headed out the door.

"Are you hungry?" he questioned back.

"No, not really. I guess we should have eaten before the treatment. Don't get me wrong. I feel fine I'm just not hungry. You should eat something, though."

"I'm not hungry either. I am ready to go home too."

The sun was shining. The snow was gone. There was a touch of spring in the air. We left Billings grateful we wouldn't have to be back soon. It was time to move forward—to get on with things as normal as possible.

I accepted the fact I had been diagnosed with cancer and the result was I had one breast. I got that. I also understood I was going to have chemo treatments once a week for one year. Bring it on! It was my decision to choose life and with every decision you make, there are consequences in that choice. I was looking forward. I wanted some normalcy back in my life including going back to work. I think Leon did too. We spent the trip home talking about things we wanted to get done in the spring. We made such big plans. The question was—were we going to get it done? Only time would tell.

Acceptance is not submission; it is acknowledgment of the facts of a situation. Then deciding what you're going to do about it.

—Kathleen Casey Theisen

Chapter Eight
If It's Not One Thing, It's Another

The first thing I did was purchased a monthly planner with a calendar. I opened it to February 27, wrote 52 beside it, and then crossed it out. I did the same thing on March 6, only I wrote 51 and crossed it out. I had completed two treatments. I continued to write descending numbers each week until I reached number 1. According to my calculations my last treatment would be the week of February 22. My intention was to cross out each number as I had a treatment. It was a visual aide to help me see the end of my chemotherapy protocol. I remember reading about a woman who would visualize each injection as something like the "pac-man" video game. As each dose was administered she pictured it eating away all the cancer cells. I tried to visualize it like that, but it didn't work for me. The calendar was a much better option.

The second thing I did was call Dr. Shorn's office to set up my next chemo treatment. I decided I wanted to have my treatments on Friday. As Leon and I had discussed I wanted to continue to work. I figured if I had my treatments on Friday and if I happened to get sick I could recover over the weekend and hopefully be ready to go back to work on Monday. The only glitch was I knew in the fall Kelly would be playing volleyball and usually her games were on Fridays and it was important for me to go to her volleyball games. So I figured when the time came I could go to the volleyball game and then have my treatment afterwards. After all I didn't know how many more I would get to see. I realized how precious my time was and I didn't take anything for granted anymore. I didn't want to miss a thing.

Dr. Shorn approved the treatment for Friday. The plan was every Friday morning before I went to work I would go to the hospital lab to have blood drawn. They would test it for my red and white blood count and have the results ready by Friday evening. It was my understanding I had to maintain a certain level of red and white blood cells before I could have chemo. Then Friday after work I would stop at the hospital for my treatment and afterwards I would drive home. It sounded like a good plan.

I was so proud. Every once in a while the demons would try to sneak into my thoughts but I held them at bay. I had everything under control. I was amazed at how well I handled the third and fourth treatments. I wasn't having any of the awful side effects. I wasn't getting sick to my stomach. I didn't have any tingling feelings in my fingers or feet. I didn't have any mouth sores and more importantly I didn't notice any significant hair loss. There wasn't anything unusual at all in fact the whole process was going really well. I was getting quite arrogant about the whole thing. I thought because I made this so-called decision to take control of the situation, I was really in control. And then reality hit and it hit hard. There is a saying that the only certainty in life is change. Well, things began to change and quickly at that.

It began on Monday morning after my fifth treatment. I woke up to get ready for work as usual. I got up and started to make the bed when I noticed a fair amount of my hair laying the pillow. The sight of it rocked my world. I was stunned. My heart fell. My stomach turned. I was afraid to touch my head for fear more hair would fall out and I was petrified to look in the mirror.

I was confused. How could I wake up one morning and find bunches of hair lying on my pillow? There was hardly anything there yesterday. I couldn't believe my eyes. I slowly bent down and gathered the strands all together. I wanted to cry. I held the fallen tresses tenderly in my hand just staring at it. I didn't know what to do. I was not emotionally prepared to deal with losing my hair.

"Good morning." Leon said, entering the bedroom. He stopped. "What's wrong?" he asked.

I held out my hand filled with my hair. He looked at it and then at me. He didn't know what to say.

"Is there a big chunk missing from my head?" I asked tentatively.
He walked over and looked over my head.

"No, in fact you can't tell there is any missing," he answered.

"Leon, don't lie to me," I said angrily extending my hand out to him.
"I am holding a handful of my hair, and you are honestly telling me you
cannot tell!"

"Honest, Candace, you cannot tell you are missing any hair."

I turned towards the mirror. I didn't know what to expect, but I
knew I was not ready to see a bald head. Thankfully Leon was right.
You could not tell I had lost any hair. I breathed a big sigh of relief. I
cautiously reached up and touched my hair. Again my stomach turned
sour as I watched a few strands float to the floor. I fought hard to keep
the tears back. Leon was unsure of what to say or do. He just stood
there waiting for me to make the next move. The sounds of dishes in
the kitchen broke the moment. Kelly and Chris were getting
themselves breakfast. I took a deep breath and turned to Leon.

"I need a hug," I said.

He opened his arms and moved closer to me. I moved in closer, and
he let me hang onto him. I held back the tears.

"I was hoping beyond hope that I wouldn't lose my hair," I said
against his shoulder.

"I know," he answered back.

"I'm going to call Billie. I am going to get my hair cut short. I want
a style that I don't have to do much with. I hope the less I have to work
with it the less hair will fall out," I said, pulling away.

"That sounds good," he said, still unsure of what to do.

I looked at him and smiled. "I'm okay. It was such a shock to see
my hair lying on the pillow. Like I said, I hoped that it wouldn't happen.
It was such a surprise. You know me; I hate surprises."

Still unsure of what to say or do, he asked, "Are you going to work
today?"

"Yes, but I don't think I'll wash my hair. It will look okay, won't
it?" I asked looking at him for reinforcement.

"It will look fine."

Leon and I carried on with our normal morning routine. The children left for their designated locations. They didn't mention they had noticed anything different about my hair. I was relieved. Leon left shortly after the children. I took one last look in the mirror before I headed out. I gingerly put a few strands in place and then sprayed it with hairspray, hoping that it would stay.

It was going to be a long day. I knew I was going to worry endlessly about whether handfuls of hair would be falling out in front of everyone. *The demons were back and up to their evil ways. They were painting an ugly picture of huge clumps of hair falling to the ground leaving large bald spots. People were pointing and laughing hysterically at the sight.* I shook them off. I needed to stay focused.

I got to work and immediately called Billie. Billie was one of the girls as well as my hairdresser. It was Monday and her day off, but I was in panic mode. I needed to do something, and I needed to do it right now.

"Hello," she answered the phone. I could tell by the tone of her voice she was either in bed still or had barely gotten up. Billie loved to sleep in on her days off.

"You have to cut my hair today," I demanded.

"Today?" she asked.

"You have to cut my hair today." I repeated the demand.

"What time?"

"I have a meeting at 9:00 for about an hour. I will be over shortly after that," I stated emphatically.

"Good. That will give me time to pee and at least have one cup of coffee," she said lightly. "You know I don't guarantee what a haircut will look like until I have at least one cup of coffee. What's up?" she asked on a more serious note.

"Oh, Billie, my hair is starting to fall out," I said trying to choke back the tears. I was at work and had to get control of myself.

"Okay, I'll see you when you get here," she said quietly.

"Thanks, Billie." Nothing more needed to be said. We said our goodbyes. I went to my meeting anxiously waiting for it to be over. I couldn't shake the feeling that strands of hair were falling all around me. The demons were working their magic. Finally the meeting concluded. I couldn't get out of there fast enough. I signed myself out and headed for Billie's house. For some reason I had it in my mind that once I had short hair it would stop falling out. It was a foolish thought, I know. But it gave me hope.

I arrived at Billie's house and walked right in without knocking on the door. She was sitting at the kitchen table still in her pajamas. She smiled.

"Want some coffee?" she asked standing up and pulling a chair out for me to sit on.

"No thanks."

She gently touched my hair. "How short do you want to go?" she asked. I wore my hair about two inches below my shoulder.

"Short," I answered.

"Candace, are you sure you want to go short?" she asked as she placed the cape around my neck.

"Billie I want to go short. If you are not willing to do it I will find someone who will," I said forcefully.

She placed her hand on my shoulder and gave it a light squeeze. "Candace, I will cut your hair short. I just don't want you to regret getting it cut short."

Tears welled up in my eyes. "I'm sorry, Billie. I have to tell you, finding a handful of my hair on my pillow this morning has knocked me for a loop. I am hoping if I get my hair cut short I won't have to touch it very much, and then it won't fall out as fast. Wishful thinking, huh?" I said as I continued to fight back the tears.

"Short it is then," she said, smiling. She grabbed her scissors and skillfully cut my strands from medium length to just above the ears. I have had medium-to-long hair since I was ten years old with one exception. I had gotten my hair cut short when Twiggy, an English model, took the U.S. by storm in the late '60s. I am not sure what possessed me to think I would look anything like Twiggy, but I tried. I failed miserably and have not had short hair since...until now.

She brushed the cut hair from my neck and handed me a mirror. I wasn't sure what I was expecting. I closed my eyes as I grabbed the mirror from her hand. I took a deep breath and held it up so I could see the new me. I was pleasantly surprised. It didn't look that bad. I could live with it.

Forgetting why I wanted it cut in the first place I reached up and ran my fingers through the bangs. A few loosened strands clung to my fingers, and I immediately put my hands down.

"You should be able to just wash it and let it dry." Billie said as she swept up the hair off the floor.

"Thank you, Billie. I really appreciate this." I felt slightly relieved it was over.

"You know you have options if you lose your hair," she said broaching the subject.

"I know. I pray every night that I won't lose it. You know there is a chance I may not lose it all, and I haven't given up hope," I said.

"Well, if you do start to lose your hair and it becomes noticeable, come down to the shop and look at some wigs. The wigs they make today are not your mother's wigs, Candace. They are really nice. If you get a good one it will be hard to tell you are wearing one."

"I know, but it's the principle of the thing. I am not ready to accept the fact that I *may* lose my hair," I said stubbornly.

"Well, the other option is a turban. We have those in stock too," she said as she poured herself another cup of coffee. "Are you sure you don't want a cup?"

"Yeah, I have to get back to work. Again, thank you," I said as I readied to leave. She grabbed me and gave me a hug.

"We gotta get together and play scrabble one of these days," she said as she let go. We loved to play scrabble, but it seemed in the past couple of years we had gotten busy doing other things.

"We really should," I said. But we both knew it wouldn't be soon.

"Love ya," she said as I walked out the door.

"Back at ya, and thanks again."

Over the next few months my hair continued to thin but I never did lose it all. People who didn't know me assumed I had very thin and fine hair. I hate to admit it but hair loss was one of the most difficult challenges I had to overcome and I am not sure why. I am not a vain person. I wear little or no makeup and spend very little time on my hair. But it did bother me. It was terribly difficult to see so much of my hair when I swept the floor. If there would have been a shedding contest between Katie the cat and me, I would have won!

As strange as this may sound, I cried more over the loss of my hair than I did my breast. Sometimes after sweeping the floor and seeing the pile of hair in the dust pan, the tears would flow freely.

Dr. Twill had told me that hair follicles are the first to resist chemotherapy and finally after five months or so my hair stopped falling out. I had heard sometimes it would grow back thicker and sometimes curly. I was hoping for a few waves or curls. But it grew back straight and that was okay with me. I was just happy it grew back.

My friend Rita says she will never forget how determined I would be about not losing all my hair. I don't know if I really got to chose that but I know I prayed passionately that I wouldn't lose it all. I was grateful God answered my prayers.

* * * * * * * * * * * * *

Around the seventh treatment my veins began to collapse. The nurse would stick the needle in, and immediately the vein would flatten out. She would have to remove the needle and try again. Sometimes it took three or four times before she would find a vein that would hold up. It got old real fast!

Dr. Shorn recommended a central catheter or port-a-cath for easier access. He assured me it only required out-patient surgery. Basically the surgeon implants a port (a small titanium reservoir with a rubber "stopper") under the skin just below the collarbone. It is attached to a tube that has been treaded through a vein and is not noticeable except for a small lump. In order to use the catheter, the nurse locates the port, cleans the area, and sticks a special needle through the skin and into the port. The chemo is then administered through the port. The good news is there would be no more if-at-first-you-don't-succeed-try-try-again sticks on my arm or hand. It sounded like a reasonable solution to me, and I agreed and had the port-a-cath put in.

I did the normal routine on Friday; blood drawn in the morning and chemo after work. I was told the nurse could use the port-a-cath immediately. However there was one little tidbit of information someone failed to mention to me or most likely I didn't hear, and that was the procedure for inserting the special needle through the skin into the port. I don't remember anyone mentioning how tender and sensitive the skin is around the collarbone area. And to make matters worse this was a new experience for the nurse as well! She had never used a port-a-cath either.

I managed not to scream out as the needle pierced the skin. And it was quite a surprise to both of us when we discovered she had to apply significant pressure to get the needle into the port. I have to admit my first thoughts were not very pleasant. I could not imagine going through this every time I had to have a treatment. I would rather have had a dozen sticks in my hand or arm than do this again. It hurt!

Fortunately Dr. Shorn had been doing his rounds and stopped in to see how the procedure went. "I see you are using the port-a-cath. How did it go?" The question was directed at the nurse.

"Fairly well, I think, although it was a little difficult to get the needle into the port," she said.

Excuse me...did she say, "a little difficult?" I thought furiously.

"How are you doing, Candace?" he said turning his attention to me.

"It hurt," I stated matter of factly.

He smiled. "Soon you will develop a callous over the port, and eventually it won't hurt anymore," he said examining the area. "This should work nicely for you."

"You promise?" I asked. I was feeling a little better about the whole thing since the pain was over.

"Just give it a couple more times," he said. I smiled back at him. I appreciated his warm bedside manner.

"In the long run your veins will thank you," he commented as he left the room.

"I guess I could tolerate a little pain as long as I know its coming, and I know there will be an end to it," I thought as I left the hospital.

Unfortunately I was unable to test that theory. I had one more treatment without incident and then things went from bad to worse. At the next treatment the nurse inserted the needle and began to administer the chemo, but it would not go into the port. She tried again and again, but the liquid would flow into the port. Finally she gave up and called Dr. Lowe, the surgeon.

I waited patiently for him to arrive. I couldn't believe this was happening. Things seemed to be going fairly well, and then of all a sudden nothing seemed to be going right at all. I could hardly wait to see what the next ten months had in store for me.

"Hi, I hear there is a problem with the port," he said, examining the area. He tried to dispense the chemo, too, but to no avail. He immediately ordered an x-ray. He didn't understand what was happening any more than the nurse did.

I walked down to the lab and they were waiting for me. It didn't take long. I went back upstairs to the waiting room and waited.

"Dr. Lowe, call *15," echoed through the building. "Dr. Lowe, call *15. I hoped that it was the results from the x-ray. I continued to wait calmly. It wasn't long before Dr. Lowe came to the waiting room.

"Just as I suspected," he said as he sat down in the chair next to me. "There is a blood clot. You are going to have to be admitted into the hospital immediately."

I looked at him in amazement. "Excuse me?" I said in total surprise.

"We must dissolve it before it moves."

I was in shock. "Can I at least go home and get some things?" I asked trying to digest everything that was happening.

"No," he said firmly. "I want to get you started on coumadin as soon as possible." He looked at me, and I must have had a confused look on my face, again. "Coumadin is used in treating blood clots, and it's important that we begin treating it immediately."

I could tell in his voice he was very concerned about the clot.

"Blood clots are rare, but obviously it happens. I don't want to take any chances," he said as he stood up. "Candace I want to get you started on coumadin now. I'll make the arrangements." He turned and walked away, leaving me speechless. I sat there trying to decide if I should call Leon first or get checked in and then call him.

"Candace" a nurse said interrupting my thoughts. "Come with me. Dr. Lowe wants an IV started."

I stood up still in a daze. *I guess that answers my question as to what I should do first,* I thought. I followed the nurse to my new accommodations. She gave me a gown. I had barely undressed when she returned with an IV unit.

"Do you mind if I sit in the chair?" I asked. I wasn't in the mood to get into bed quite yet.

"No problem. I guess since the port is blocked it's back to finding a vein," she said as she reached for my right arm.

I pulled it away and extended my left hand. "I was told not to let anyone stick a needle in my right arm." I said. "I had surgery on my right side."

"It's been a while since you had surgery. I'm sure it would be okay."

"Whatever.... I want you to use my left arm." I said firmly. She didn't say anymore about it. She tied a rubber strap around my arm and searched for a vein that might work. It only took three or four times before she found a vein that didn't collapse. She gently inserted the needle, capped the port, and removed the strap. She attached the IV and monitored it until it started a steady drip.

"Dr. Lowe has ordered coumadin for you, and as soon as it comes up I will bring it in. In the meantime I give you your chemo," she announced. Slowly she administered each dose. When she was through she rechecked the monitor and left the room. I continued to sit in the chair in a fog. I couldn't believe I was in the hospital again. *Well, I guess the bright side to this mess is another treatment is out of the way,* I thought optimistically.

Finally I came to my senses and called Leon. He was shocked. I assured him I wasn't sick and this was a precautionary measure. He said he would be up as soon as he changed his clothes plus he would let everyone know I was in the hospital…again. I didn't want him to but I knew if anyone found out I was in the hospital and didn't call them, they would be hurt. And it's a good thing he did call everyone! I spent the next four days in the hospital bored to tears. It was nice when someone came to visit because it helped the time pass so much quicker.

Ron and Judy stopped by one evening. They asked their questions and I answered them to the best of my ability and then we talked about much happier things. Ron started reminiscing about the time we had gone over to Rita and Larry's for a neighborhood barbeque. There were about thirty people gathered. A group of us were sitting on the back deck laughing and telling stories. Being the good host she was Rita came out to see how we were doing. She stood by the patio screen door observing the activities and making sure our cups were full!

Larry had just begun telling us a story about a delivery man who had ran over a cat. The man was devastated and felt he needed to tell the owner. He went to the nearest house and asked the woman who answered the door if she owned a cat. The woman said yes. The man proceeded to tell her he had just run over a cat. The woman asked, "What did the cat look like when you hit it?"

Immediately Larry threw his arms back in the air and put a shocked look on his face! The action took us all by surprise, and we laughed. Rita looked slightly puzzled for a moment and then her face lit up as she got it. We laughed more.

Now not to be outdone Rita had a story too. She began telling us about going home to see her sisters. She had seven of them! Can you imagine…eight girls under one roof! Anyhow, they were all together sitting on the patio drinking, laughing and having a great time when one of her sisters got up to go into the house. She was so busy talking she didn't notice the screen door was closed and walked right into it. Rita buckled over with laughter. We laughed too. Then she continued to tell us her sister hit the screen so hard her nose left a dent in it. Rita could hardly contain herself. We were laughing but I think more with Rita than we were about the story!

Finally satisfied her guests were entertained Rita turned to go into the house and bam…ran right smack dab into the screen door. She hit it so hard it threw her back a couple of steps! But the best part was the dent in the screen from her nose! We laughed uncontrollably. There was not a dry eye in the place.

Ron, Judy, Leon and I were enjoying reliving the moment so much the nurse came and closed the door. We couldn't help ourselves. It was just too funny! We laughed until our sides hurt but it felt so good to laugh.

And then it was time for them to go.

* * * * * * * * * * * * *

I was released on Tuesday, and none too soon! Dr. Lowe was not ready to remove the port-a-cath yet, because he wanted to try it one more time. He was going to administer it this time to make sure everything was working properly. At the moment that was Plan A.

Friday arrived, and as usual I had my blood drawn in the morning, and after work I went to the hospital for my treatment. Dr. Lowe was anxiously waiting. He cleaned the area and proceeded to stick the needle through my skin and into the port.

"Hopefully this work will today," Dr. Lowe stated as he diligently tried to push the needle through to the port. It hurt. I had not developed a callous over the area as of yet. I tried not to flinch, but it was difficult.

"Okay, I'm through!" he exclaimed happily. I did not have the same feelings. I was still pouting over the fact I had to endure pain. I didn't figure it was part of the bargain.

Now I wish I could say that the port-a-cath worked, but it didn't. Dr. Lowe tried three or four times and still was unable to get the chemo through the port. I was quite finished with this whole process. It was time to try Plan B!

Dr. Lowe called Dr. Shorn, and they came up with Plan B. Plan B was to remove the central port-a-cath and insert a Groshong catheter. The Groshong catheter is a tunneled catheter. The surgeon takes one end of a tube and threads it about six inches under the skin on the chest. The other end dangles out, making it available for immediate use. Although I wasn't terribly excited about a tube hanging from my chest I knew the port-a-cath needed to go. I was told the only possible side effect of the tunneled catheter was a chance of bacterial infection. However the chances were slim. I decided to try it. It was an out-patient procedure, and it seemed like a good plan. I had the Groshong catheter inserted.

Although the upkeep of the Groshong was a nuisance it worked like a charm. I could have my blood drawn through it and the chemo administered into it—no pain and needle sticks. I couldn't have been happier except for one little thing...the side-effects from the prednisone.

* * * * * * * * * * * *

Dr. Twill had started me on a fairly high dose of prednisone with a gradual reduction over a period of seventy days. Prednisone is a steroid and as with any medication has a long list of side effects. I had been taking it for about thirty days or so when some of the side-effects kicked in.

First I developed what I learned is commonly referred to as steroid acne and cushingold or moon face. My face was as round as the moon and I mean perfectly round! It was so strange to look at myself in the mirror. It did not look like me at all! And then to top it off I had pimples everywhere! I also experienced blurred vision which Dr. Twill thought may be related to the prednisone as well. But that was the least of it. I gained twenty-five pounds! I was not happy about that at all. I had so hoped to lose weight not gain it.

Another side effect is a "false sense of well-being." I didn't understand what that meant until I finished the prescription.

For the most part while I was taking prednisone I felt pretty good. Besides the emotional turmoil on losing my hair, weight gain and my veins collapsing, I was handling the chemo quite well.

I had finished my twelfth treatment and the last of the prednisone around the middle of May. All was well. But you know the saying, "All good things must come to an end."

Up to this point I had been driving myself to the hospital and home after my treatment. And then one day, out of the blue, I got sick. At first I was able to drive home and run to the bathroom before I started to…how do I put it politely? In simple terms, throw-up! Soon I would make it only to the parking lot and lose everything before I got into the car. Then I managed to get to the visitor's bathroom in the waiting room. I was always worried someone would hear me because I was sure the awful sound from my vomiting was resonating through the halls. I always hoped no one was in the waiting room when I left.

It didn't take long before I could only manage to make it to the bathroom in the room where I had my chemo, and finally I simply resorted to the garbage pail.

I reached the point that when Friday came around I would get sick to my stomach even before I had the treatment. It was awful. Dr. Twill ordered a "Benadryll cocktail" to help with the nausea. I tried it a couple of times, but didn't like how I felt so I refused to take it.

There was quite commotion the first time I refused to take it. The nurse didn't know what to do. So she called Dr. Shorn to inform him that I wouldn't take the medicine. He was surprised, too, but told her it was my choice. I was glad he agreed, because I had enough on my plate without arguing about whether or not I was going to take the medicine. I was determined not to take it.

However I have to admit I am not sure it was a good choice. Over the next months I continued to get sicker. In fact I dubbed myself, "Vomit Queen of Glendive." The dry-heaves were the worst. Sometimes I would wake up in the middle of the night gagging and begin to vomit until there wasn't anything left to get rid of. In the beginning I would rush to the bathroom but I wised up and kept a bucket beside the bed.

I felt bad for Leon. One night during a dry-heave episode I asked him, "How I could I possibly be throwing up when there wasn't anything left to come up?"

He didn't say a word. What could he say? I know he felt so helpless. When I had finished and returned to bed he would gently hold me in his arms. It was very comforting. I snuggled in close until…the hot flash hit!

* * * * * * * * * * * * *

The hot flashes began shortly after my stint in the hospital with the port-a-cath. During my stay I had my menstrual period and I am happy to report it was the last time I had it. Pre-menopausal symptoms were one of the side effect s from chemo.

In the beginning it seemed I had a hot flash about every five to ten minutes and I am not exaggerating! I would barely get over one and another one would start. The worst ones were the ones that started at the bottom of my spine and I could feel the heat work its way up. The higher it moved up the spine, the hotter I became. Sometimes I would feel edgy and antsy. I felt like I wanted to crawl out of my skin. But those were nothing compared to the night sweats, wow!

Before cancer we had a heating blanket on our bed. In the winter when it was so cold, Leon or I would turn it on about an hour before we went to bed so when we got into bed it was nice and toasty. Then the hot flashes began and the heating blanket became history real fast! Typically I went to bed before Leon so by the time he got to bed I had it pretty warmed up. He didn't miss the heating blanket either!

Although the hot flashes were an inconvenience—especially when I had one, two and sometimes three or more during a business meeting—I figured in the scheme of things it was something I could handle. I can honestly say there has not been one month that has gone by when I thought, *Gee, I miss having my period.* I don't miss anything about the bloating, bleeding, or mood-swings. It was the one side effect I appreciated! It was the chills and fevers that became almost intolerable.

* * * * * * * * * * * * *

The Groshong catheter worked great for about the next six months, and then in the middle of December things began to change. I continued to have my blood drawn every Friday morning. Since I had started getting sick I would go home after work, and Leon would drive me to the hospital.

The change was subtle at first. I would have my blood drawn and go back to work as usual. But as the day wore on I began to feel ill, but in a different kind of way. I felt this chill deep inside my bones. I think I have mentioned once or twice I hate being cold. I thought it was just another side effect from the chemo, so I didn't put too much thought into it. But then one day it hit me hard.

I had had my blood drawn as usual, and on my way back to work this terrible feeling came over me. I was cold, very, very cold deep inside my bones. I headed home instead and by the time I reached the house I was so cold my teeth were chattering uncontrollably. I struggled to get into the house. I realized it was December, and it was cold outside, but this was a totally different kind of cold. I grabbed the heaviest blanket I could find and the heating pad which I turned to high. My teeth were chattering so hard they began to hurt. All I knew is that I wanted to warm up and warm up fast. It was awful. I lay huddled in a blanket with the heating pad on high and my teeth chattering for about an hour when finally I began to warm up. The problem was I went from freezing cold to a temperature of 104 degrees! I didn't know what to do. I knew a temperature this high was not good and that I had to get the fever down. I managed to get a couple of Tylenol down. I also knew I shouldn't wrap myself back up in the blanket but having the fever felt so much better than having the chills. I couldn't help myself. Warm was much better than cold. I think I mentioned I hated being cold!

By the time Leon had got home in the afternoon I had managed to get my temperature down to 101 degrees. We headed to hospital as usual. I informed the nurse I had had chills and a fever earlier in the day. She took my temp and it registered 101 degrees. She called Dr. Shorn. He told her I could not have chemo as long as I had a fever. At first I was elated I didn't have to have chemo. But then it dawned on me that without chemo I was defenseless and there was a chance the cancer would return. I definitely didn't want that to happen. I was confused and fearful. I ended up spending the entire weekend fighting with the demons instead of enjoying not being sick from the chemo. I couldn't wait until next Friday. I preferred the chemo rather than dealing with the demons.

I continued to have chills and fever through December, January and the first two weeks in February. Dr. Shorn consulted with Dr. Twill and they decided if my temperature stayed around 100 to 101 degrees I could have my treatment. I missed a total of four treatments all together.

My last treatment was February 22. I had mixed emotions about the whole thing. On one hand I was thrilled, excited, happy—all those adjectives that describe complete joy. I was finally done with chemotherapy. I was tired of the vomiting, chills, fevers, tingling in my fingers and bottoms of my feet and the weight gain. But on the other hand I felt vulnerable. I had no weapons to defend myself against this dreadful disease.

The only limit in our realization of tomorrow will be our doubts of today. Let us move forward with strong and active faith.

—Franklin Delano Roosevelt

Chapter Nine
You Don't Have to Do It Alone

"I can't do this by myself. I need to meet people who have survived. I need to talk to people who won their battle with this awful disease. I need to meet that person who has lost her hair, and it has grown back. I need to know there really is a light at the end of this tunnel!"

* * * * * * * * * * * * *

The first person I went to talk to was Dan. He was general manager of the smallest TV station in the nation! It was a real asset for Glendive. Not only was Dan our local radio and TV celebrity, he was the local sports announcer. Everyone in the area knew Dan, and everyone liked him too.

Dan had been diagnosed with testicular cancer ten years before me. I found out Dan had cancer through his wife Carol. Carol, Judy, and I bowled on Wednesday night. We all lived in the neighborhood, so we carpooled. Imagine that! One Wednesday night on our way to the bowling alley, Carol told us that Dan hadn't been feeling very well. She tried to convince him to go to the doctor, but as is typical with a man, he was reluctant to do so. She was getting very concerned because he kept feeling worse and worse. Finally she convinced him to go...and he was diagnosed with cancer. And it had spread. He went on an all-out war to save his life!

What I admired most about Dan was his willingness to share his ordeal at the time when you didn't talk openly about cancer. There were still a lot of unknown's and a stigma about cancer. Would you believe some people thought you could catch cancer by being around someone who had it! It was their generation's AIDS.

However, instead of hiding it Dan took it to the airways. He went on a local TV program called "Let's Talk About It." It was a half hour show that featured community happenings, and it aired every Sunday night.

I remember watching it at the time and thinking how courageous he was to share something that most people kept a secret especially something like testicular cancer. I remember him telling how at one point his veins had collapsed except in his little finger. It was the only place they could draw blood from anymore. I couldn't appreciate the enormity of that at the time, but I certainly could relate to it now.

"Hi, Dan, are you busy?" I said, lightly tapping on his office door.

"Hello, Candace, how are you?" he asked as he rose and extended his hand. "Come on in."

"Thanks," I said as I sat down. "I know you are busy, but I need a moment of your time. I am not sure if you heard, but I was recently diagnosed with breast cancer."

"I heard, and I'm sorry. How are you doing?" he asked, genuinely concerned.

"Okay, I guess. I've been frustrated with some of the side effects of the chemo."

"I can appreciate that." He smiled.

"I decided I needed to talk with people who have been through it. So I think I'm going to try to start a cancer-support group. I'm thinking we would meet once a month and maybe do some educational stuff, but the major focus would be sharing what we are going through. What do you think?"

"I think it's a great idea. You should talk to Shirley. If I remember correctly she was diagnosed with breast cancer last year. She might have some good ideas," he offered.

"Do you think you would come?" I asked.

"I might attend from time to time, but not all the time. I have a pretty busy schedule," he said. "However the station will do PSAs [public service announcements], and when you are ready I encourage you to do 'Let's Talk About It.' And," he said as he took a deep sigh, "I have to be honest; if I have any spare time I like to be home."

"Thanks, I appreciate that. Do you think the community will be open to it?"

"Absolutely, and I think you will find a person will come depending on where they are with the disease. In the early stages they may need more support, but as they get better they may not need as much. Unfortunately, you will probably always have new people coming."

"I suppose so," I said, nodding in full agreement. "I have one more question to ask, and then I'll let you get back to work. Dan, how did you handle the treatment? Does the fear of cancer ever leave you?"

"There were many times I didn't think I could handle the treatment. But you have two choices: never give up hope, or give up and die. I never gave up hope. And as far as living with the fear of cancer, each day it gets a little better. I don't worry about it much anymore. I do, however, regret waiting so long before going to the doctor. It would have saved me a lot of pain and agony if it would have been detected early. Anyway, I have been told I probably won't die of cancer but from the treatment. There was significant damage done to my heart, but I don't dwell on that much either. I am amazed at how far medicine has come since I was diagnosed. The chemo I received then and what they use now are totally different, and thank goodness! Through it all I learned a couple of things, and my best advice to you is get rid of all the garbage," he said sitting back in his chair.

"What do you mean by getting rid of the garbage?" I asked.

"Use your energy to fight the disease. If you have any hate in your heart, let it go. If you have stress in your life, find a way to relax. Don't spend another minute thinking negatively. Use your energy positively," he said as the phone rang. "I hope that makes sense."

"Yes, and you take the call. I'll keep in touch," I said as I rose to leave. I waved and mouthed a "thank you" as I left his office.

Dan attended the support group one or two times. True to his word, the TV and radio station aired PSAs regularly. I eventually did "Let's Talk About It." In fact I was a featured guest three or four times. And he was right. Each day the fear of cancer lessened.

* * * * * * * * * * * *

Some people come into our lives and quickly go. Some stay for a while and leave footprints on our hearts. And we are never, ever the same.

—Anonymous

I had left Dan's office and went directly over to Shirley's office. She was the director of the Domestic Violence program. Like Dan, Shirley was well known in the community for her generosity and kindness. I knew who Shirley was but had never been formally introduced to her. Shirley and her family attended the same church as we did.

I lightly tapped on the door. "Hi, Shirley, do you have a minute?" I asked as I peeked my head into the room.

She looked up from her work and immediately smiled. Shirley had the kind of smile that lit up a room. It was a genuine smile that touched her lips and sparkled through her eyes. It was the kind of smile that you are naturally drawn to. "Candace, of course. Come on in," she said exuberantly. "How are you?"

"I am doing good, thank you. I have a couple of questions for you," I said sitting down. "I just left Dan's office at the TV station, and he suggested that I visit with you. So here I am."

"How are you doing?" she asked with genuine concern.

I could tell from the tone in her voice she knew I had been diagnosed with cancer. "I have good days, and I have bad days. I think that is the protocol for the disease and the treatment," I said smiling. She nodded.

"The reason I am here is I want to start a cancer support group," I said. "I wish I could say it was for unselfish reasons, but I need to meet and talk with people who have lost their hair, and it has grown back."

She quickly glanced at my thinning hair, and then her eyes returned to mine. "I think that is a wonderful idea. What do you have in mind?"

"I thought maybe we would meet once a month. Maybe do some educational things. But the focus of the meeting would be sharing what you are going through at the moment."

"Sounds good. We could also bring in a speaker. I could contact the hospital to see if one of the doctors or nurses would be willing to come once in a while," she added.

"Does that mean you would be willing to help me?" I asked.

"Of course. I think it is a wonderful idea. I know of at least seven or eight people right now who would attend. When and where do you think would be a good time to meet?"

"I was thinking Thursday night at 7:00 p.m., but I don't know where. Do you have any ideas?"

"There is a meeting room at the clinic. I'll see what I need to do to reserve it. How soon do you want to meet?" she said as she was making notes.

"Let's shoot for next Thursday. You can check on the room. Once we have everything confirmed I'll get a hold of Dan. He said the station would do some PSAs. I will also talk to someone at the newspaper. I know the paper runs a calendar of events. Later on they may be willing to do a story."

"I'll let you know as soon as I get information on the room."

"Thanks, Shirley, for helping me. I really appreciate it," I said as I stood to leave. She rose from her chair and came around the desk. She placed her hand lightly on my arm as we walked to the door. It was a reassuring gesture.

"Candace, I think a cancer support group is a great idea. I am more than willing to help," she said. And so our friendship began.

* * * * * * * * * * * * *

"Shirley, can I ask you a question?" I asked as we were driving to our first cancer support group meeting.

"Of course," she said.

"How did you handle losing your hair?" I asked.

"I didn't lose my hair," she said. "I found my lump very early through a mammogram. It was small, so I was fortunate; all I had to have was the surgery. I didn't need chemo or radiation."

I was taken aback! I didn't know what to say. All I could muster was, "Really!"

She continued, "It was discovered when I had my annual checkup and mammogram. I chose to have surgery and reconstruction immediately."

Again, all I could think of to say—at least out loud—was, "Really!" I am ashamed to admit it but my first reaction was, *How could she possibly understand what it is like to have chemo or radiation when she hadn't been through it?* I was disappointed that she had not gone through all the "yuk" associated with the treatment. I had this lovely picture in my mind of her and me sharing stories about vomiting, hair loss, and weight gain. And now I come to find out she hadn't been through any of it! Personally her cancer didn't count! I changed the subject and started talking about the meeting. We finished the rest of trip discussing the agenda.

I was amazed as one person after another filled the room. By the time the meeting was scheduled to begin there were twelve of us all together. I was surprised at all the different ages, but not surprised it was all women. We introduced ourselves and announced the type of cancer each of us had or had gone through. Although the majority of us had breast cancer there was a mixed bag of cancers. There was non-Hodgkin's lymphoma, liver, and lung cancer. I watched each one as they talked about their disease and the treatment. Some just had surgery (like Shirley), some had gone through or were going through chemo, some through radiation, and some didn't have any treatment options at all. The end result was we all had one thing in common…none of us were ready to give up.

But the most important thing I learned that evening was about my friend Shirley. I discovered that she had this wonderful gift. She had this great capacity to listen. It went beyond hearing the words everyone said. It was her strength to absorb it and make it her own. I soon realized Shirley may not have gone through the "yuk," but her selfless compassion and understanding of human tragedy was amazing. It became very clear to me why people were immediately drawn to her. Shirley authentically cared about you. There were no pretenses it was simply her way.

The cancer support group continued to meet once a month for the next two years. Shirley and I took turns getting speakers and such, in other words, food. I remember someone telling me you can have a terrible meeting but if the food is good, no one will remember how bad the meeting was! At one point The American Cancer Society had contacted me and asked if we were interested in doing "I Can Cope."

"I Can Cope" is an educational program to help people go through cancer with the least amount of trauma. It runs for about eight weeks. It is a very good program, and I highly recommend it if you have the chance to go. I recommend the book too.

I also discovered Dan was right. There was always someone new to the group. Some of the original twelve attended faithfully, and some didn't. And on a rare occasion a man would show up. We never knew how many would be there, and it didn't matter. Once you stepped into the room you were connected. I believe that everyone understood, no matter what their circumstances. There was always someone there for them.

The other interesting thing that happened was many times a caregiver would join us. Most of the time it was a child of parent who had cancer. They were as frustrated with the disease as the parent who had it. They were struggling because they didn't know what to do and for many of them the roles had been reversed. Their parent had an owie and they wanted to make it all better. They wanted to fix it. The challenge was helping them to understand they couldn't fix it.

I tried to explain it like this; typically when you are first diagnosed with cancer you are faced with your own mortality and that is very, very frightening. No matter how strong you think you are you are never prepared for it and your first thoughts are you are going to die. And when you lose someone close to you—like yourself and it doesn't get much closer than that—it is only natural to go through a grieving process.

First you are shocked. You are numb. It's hard to believe it is real. And then you go through denial. You cannot believe it is really happening to you. You know it happens to other people but not to you. You feel you are too young, have too much to do yet or not prepared to die this way. And that is when fear and hard core anger set in. You become angry and ask, "Why me?" You are very angry at God because you don't understand how He could let this happen to you.

You can get so angry you lash out at anyone who comes within arms length of you. It's difficult to overcome the, It's-not-fair—poor-me thought process. And then you finally go through the resolution process and you come to terms with it. You accept the diagnosis and deal with everything that comes with it. It is that time when you give it back to God and trust Him to help you through it no matter what the outcome. The key is going "through" each step.

I explained the most important role as care-giver is to help their loved one go through the process. But it was difficult for them to understand that patience, love and understanding were important. They wanted something more tangible. This was not the answer they were looking for, they wanted to do more.

Shirley and I talked at length about what we could offer the care-giver. Their presence helped the group understand cancer not only affected the individual but the people who loved them as well. It was an important lesson.

* * * * * * * * * * * * *

Eventually the group disbanded. It just happened. However Shirley and I continued to get together once a month for lunch. Our friendship evolved from a cancer-related relationship to personal one and it was nice. I always enjoyed her company.

One day at lunch she told me she had not been feeling well. She had developed a persistent cough. She believed she had caught a cold and just couldn't seem to get rid of it. She was also very disappointed with the fact her doctor had retired. She was having difficulty finding a new one and she was concerned because she was way past her annual physical. I understood her dilemma. I was in the same boat. Dr. Shorn had left too leaving me without a doctor. We promised each other if either one of us found a new doctor we liked we would let each other know. We said our good-byes.

It was the last time we had the opportunity to have lunch together. Shirley did find another doctor and she had her annual physical. She discovered the persistent cough was not a by-product of a cold. It was lung cancer and it had spread.

Shirley spent the next couple of months fighting for her life. She went through the whole grieving process of shock, denial, anger, and acceptance. I remember one day when I went to visit her. She was lying on the couch and she looked worn. She smiled but for the first time the smile did not reach her eyes. She held her Bible close to her. We reminisced about the support group meetings and other things in general. We sat quietly for a moment and then she softly whispered she was dying. The words took my breath away. I didn't know what to say. How do you counter with a statement like that? She held her Bible even closer to her and a look of contentment washed over her face. She trusted God with all her heart. I admired her strength.

But I was uncomfortable and I did the most cowardly thing. I made up a lame excuse and left. Why didn't I have had the courage to stay and pray with her? Why when my friend needed me did I run away? I know without a doubt she would have been there for me. It is something I have and always will regret.

I will never forget the day I received the news that Shirley had died. I was busy doing insignificant things when Rita stopped by. She had been at the hospital with the family when God called Shirley home. Rita wanted me to hear it from a friend and not through the rumor mill. I cried deeply for my friend Shirley and for me.

Shortly after Shirley and I met she had given me a gift I still have today. She had framed a canvas on which she had cross-stitched "The joy of the Lord is your strength." It is a gentle reminder of how fragile life is. But more importantly it is a steadfast reminder that I have been truly blessed to have had the honor to know Shirley and call her my friend. I think of her often. I miss my friend Shirley.

The joy of the Lord is your strength.

—Nehemiah 8:10

Chapter Ten
Faith, Love, and Laughter

When you are diagnosed with cancer it's like riding an emotional roller coaster; it takes you to great heights of despair and then…swoosh, you plummet down to deep depths of hopelessness, and then you even out and find faith and hope. And just when you think you have everything under control…you begin the ride over again!

It was a long and trying year. I remember telling Rita, "If it was only the cancer." But it seemed it was always one thing or another, between the drains, catheters, blood clots, chills, fevers, hot flashes, weight gain, and feeling sorry for myself…just to name a few, cancer was the least of my worries. But through it all, I was given the opportunity to realize at an early age life is fragile and not forever. In the scheme of things it was a small price to pay to know that each day is a blessing and I take special care with every day I have been given.

Cancer made me question my faith at times but I never lost faith and the end result is my faith has grown stronger. It is an awesome feeling knowing that you are loved by a kind and forgiving God. I get frustrated with myself at times because I know the rules and yet I continue to sin everyday. Sometimes when I sin I find myself negotiating with God. I'll pray, "God I won't do this or that anymore if you just answer this one prayer." And then, with great shame that I am admitting to this one…there are times when I ask Him to rate my sin on a scale from 1—10! In my mind I try to justify it: something between a "little white lie" and a "really big lie." However the reality is a lie is a lie, and sin is sin, and there are consequences to both.

But the real clincher is I used to think it was interesting when things went wrong in someone's life, they would blame God first. They would ask, "How can you do this to me?" I thought if you really believe how could you possibly blame God? But guess who got first in line to ask that question when diagnosed with cancer? It was me—weak, sinful me.

The good news is God is kind, forgiving and is always there to pick up the pieces. He is steadfast in his presence. I remember Shirley's unrelenting devotion to God when she knew she was dying. I on the other hand let fear take over and I ran away like a scared puppy. But Shirley didn't question whether God was with her. Like it says in the poem, "Footprints in the Sand," Shirley knew God was carrying her gently in His arms. I get goose bumps just thinking how phenomenal and unconditional that insight must be! Wow!

Cancer opened my eyes to a lot of things, but especially to all the love I have been blessed with. My mother and father who found it difficult at times to be civil to each other put their differences aside and we were able to have holiday dinners together again as a family. It was wonderful. It was really quite a sacrifice on their part and one I really appreciated.

When I wanted a diversion or wanted to play cards, we would call Ron, Judy, Rita and Larry, and they would simply ask, "When, where, and what time?" They never mentioned they were too busy or too tired.

And most of all none of my friends took anything personally. I remember one time Billie called me to see how I was doing. I had just gotten home from one of my treatments. We were visiting, and I suddenly had the urge to throw up. In the middle of her conversation I started to gag and without an explanation slammed the phone on the receiver and took care of my business. I never did call her back to let her know what happened. Later we did visit and laugh about it. She didn't know whether she should call back or wait until I called back, so neither of us did any thing, and she didn't take it personally.

Sometimes when I would get frustrated with the whole treatment process, I have to admit I would lash out at anyone who was within arm's length. There were times I didn't want to tell another soul I was doing fine. I just wanted to be left alone. Unfortunately Leon, Chris, Kelly, and my mom had to endure the brunt of most of my frustrations.

However I am very blessed because we are a close family and our love is unconditional…always. I don't ever take that blessing for granted.

One of the rules I established early on was when someone came to visit they could ask all the questions they had but then they had to make me happy and make me laugh! I figured it was a simple request and thank goodness all my friends and family took it seriously!

In fact do you know laughter has been proven to be medically therapeutic? Specialists in health care, education and business all say laughing reduces stress, builds your immune system and gives you energy. Studies also show laughter speeds your metabolism and helps you burn calories. Medical studies indicate that laughter boosts levels of endorphins, the body's natural painkillers, and suppresses levels of epinephrine, the stress hormone. To put it technically, some studies have shown the following physiological effects of laughter in the immune system alone: increase in the number and activity of T cells and natural killer cells, which attack viruses, foreign cells and cancer cells; increase in gamma interferon, a blood chemical that transmits messages in the nervous system and stimulates the immune system, a rise immunoglobulin A, an antibody that fights upper respiratory tract infections and lots, lots more. In simpler terms, "Laughter is the best medicine!"

Now I have to admit it was difficult to find things funny when you spend a lot of time hugging a toilet or sweeping up mounds of your hair on the floor! But it always felt so good to laugh.

In fact I was surprised as to the lengths my family and friends went to just to make me laugh. I have to share one final story with you. I celebrated my 38th birthday with a party. It was the middle of July, I was in the middle of chemo, and it was hot, hot, hot! I had to wear a hat, pants and long sleeves because my skin was sensitive to sunlight from the chemo. Also by now I was about twenty pounds heavier, I had tingling in my fingers and toes, and my coordination was slightly off…I always had this feeling I was going to tip over!

My guests were all in their late thirties or over forty, and none of us were in any physical condition. So the question becomes, why were we trying to play volleyball? The answer is, "I don't know." You've heard the saying, "The spirit is willing, but the body is weak"? Well, that kind of sums it up. I remember Ron forgot he was over forty, overweight, and out of shape when he jumped up to return a volley and instead landed on the ground with a thud. He lay there quietly. For a brief moment we thought he might have seriously hurt himself. When he finally rolled over, brushed the dirt from his face, shirt, and skinned knees, we tried, and I honestly mean we tried not to laugh, but it was impossible. Judy laughed so hard she peed her pants, and of course that made us laugh all the more! Now, is that not going beyond the call of duty to make your friends laugh?

There is a tire store I drive by on my way home. Every two weeks they put a different saying on the marquee. The other day I drove by, and this is what they had displayed. "My wife and I had words. I didn't get to use mine." I laughed and laughed. You may not think its funny, and that is okay. But whatever strikes your funny-bone and makes you laugh…do it!

Midge and Susan stopped by one day to see how I was doing. I was in full bloom! I had gained twenty pounds since the last time I had seen them, and they were quite surprised. I will never forget Susan saying, "This is the healthiest I have ever seen you!" I looked at her, and we laughed. I assured her it was the most polite way of saying, "You have gotten quite pleasantly plump!" I still kid her about it today.

I am forever grateful to my family and friends for the boundless tears of joy and laughter they brought into my life. I am truly blessed.

* * * * * * * * * * * *

I am proud to announce it has been seventeen years since I was first diagnosed with cancer. I just had my annual mammogram and physical. The doctor and I talked about the different treatment options available today. I am excited about the new drugs for treating nausea—although I hope I never, never have to test them! But who knows?

I will never say I am cancer free. My belief is cancer never leaves you. Every time you have a new ache or pain, the ornery little demons reappear. Don't get me wrong; I don't dwell on it or let it consume my thoughts and the good news is the thought comes and goes as quickly as it appears. But the fear of cancer returning rears its ugly head occasionally.

Sometimes I look back I think what would I have done differently. I guess I did the best I could with the information I had at the time. The lessons I learned was I wish I would have been more open with my family and friends. When we talk about it now I have discovered it was very frustrating for them because they didn't know what to do to help me. And they wanted to help—just like the care-givers who attended the support group. If I had shared more information with them it would have helped them to understand what I was going through and they would have worried much less about me. I found out they had their little demons too.

One of my biggest regrets is in the very beginning not having someone come with me to my appointments. It seemed like I only heard half of what was said and I was constantly blindsided and taken by surprise. I hate surprises. I regret thinking I could do it on my own. It would have saved me a lot of anxiety if I would have had someone with me to hear the half I was missing. Instead I never knew what was going to happen or when it was going to happen. I strongly urge you— take someone with you to take notes and ask the hard questions, please!

Every once in a while, especially after I have talked with someone who is going through cancer, I ask myself, "If I was diagnosed with cancer today would I go through treatment again, knowing what I know now?" First I have to admit I hope and pray I never have to go through it again, but yes, I would do it again. For all the regrets, frustrations and fears, I gained so much, much more.

I want to thank you for letting me share my story with you. May God be forever in your heart and bless you always.

What God Hath Promised

God hath not promised skies always blue,
Flower strewn pathways all our lives through;
God has not promised sun without rain,
Joy without sorrow, peace without pain.
But God hath promised strength for the day,
Rest for the labor, light for the way,
Grace for the trials, help from above,
Unfailing sympathy, undying love....

Amy Flint Johnson

DISCOVERING YOUR SPIRIT
Journal

The Essence of a New Day

This is the beginning of a new day.
You have been given this day to use as you will.
You can waste it or your can use it for good.
What you do today is important because you are
exchanging a day of your life for it.
When tomorrow comes, this day will be gone forever;
in its place is something that you have left behind...
let it be something good.

—Anonymous

Everyone experiences "those days." Those days are when nothing seems to go right or you feel sad. The *Discovering Your Spirit* journal is designed for "those days." Use the journal when you are struggling with a challenge. Use it as a tool to understanding yourself, others, managing stress and maintaining a fluid spirit through chaos, change and crisis. Use it as a tool to put things into perspective and keep you grounded. Use it as a sounding board when you become frustrated and angry. Use it when you are happy. Use it when you need to cry. Use it when you need a laugh. Use it to discover your many blessings. Just use it.

I have given you questions to help you get started but that doesn't mean you should limit yourself to those questions. As you go through your life there are circumstances that may confuse you so use the journal as a reference or guide to help you sort things out. Remember this is your journal there are no right or wrong answers. The journal is about how you are thinking and feeling at the moment. My only request is that you are completely honest with yourself. Always write down what is true to you—be authentic.

Vision

Your Vision of How It Was Supposed to Be

As children we had fantasies about what we wanted to be when we grew up—whether it was a doctor...lawyer...teacher...movie star...nurse...President of the United States—you could be anything you wanted to be!

As a child, what was your dream?

Dream

I Have a Dream

Think about it…if there were no obstacles in your way, what kind of house would you live in, what kind of car would you drive, what kind of career would you choose, where would you live?

If I had a great deal of money, time and talent I would:

Gratefulness

I Am Grateful For…

Sometimes when life gets hard it's difficult to find things to be grateful for. Think of it as treasure hunting. Treasure hunting is looking for positive results in negative situations.

Identify at least fifty things you are grateful for in your life, past and present. If you find more make the list longer. Refer back to the list during those times when you struggle to find something to be thankful for and never stop adding to the list.

1.
2.
3.
4.
5.
6.
7.
8.
9.
10.
11.
12.
13.
14.
15.
16.
17.
18.
19.
20.

21.

22.

23.

24.

25.

26.

27.

28.

29.

30.

31.

32.

33.

34.

35.

36.

37.

38.

39.

40.

41.

42.

43.

44.

45.

46.

47.

48.

49.

50.

51.

52.

53.

54.

55.

56.
57.
58.
59.
60.
61.
62.
63.
64.
65.
66.
67.
68.
69.
70.
71.
72.
73.
74.
75.
76.
77.
78.
79.
80.
81.
82.
83.
84.
85.
86.
87.
88.
89.
90.

91.
92.
93.
94.
95.
96.
97.
98.
99.
100.

What do I value most in my relationship with my spouse?

What do I value most in my relationship with my children?

What do I value most in my relationship with my friends?

Giving
Giving It Away with No Expectations

Why is it so difficult to give especially without expectations? Typically when we say, "Thank you," to someone we expect them to respond with, "You're welcome." Is not human nature to think that person is rude or uncaring if they don't respond? Don't we focus more on the expectation than the joy of giving?

Think about it. When you give without expectations, you give because the gift of giving brings you joy. There are no disappointments. The joy is giving not receiving and it doesn't get any better than that!

Do you give without expectations? When you give what are your expectations?

What are some ways you can give without expectations?

How do you give away time?

Do you make special time for your children?

Do you make special time for your spouse?

Do you make special time for your friends?

Do you volunteer in the community?

Although giving without expectations can bring you great joy, you must remember to give to you also. Give yourself permission to treat yourself without feeling guilty. Make a list of the things you enjoy doing…things that make you feel good. Maybe you love a hot bubble bath, a pedicure, a manicure or just some quiet time. Give yourself the gift of time to pamper yourself.

Favorite Things

Oooh...It Makes Me Feel So Good

There are events in your life that always seem to make you smile—your first kiss, the birth of your child, and possibly your most embarrassing moment! Write down your fondest memories and remember to enter the new ones when they happen.

Favorite Things

My Favorite Foods

Some favorite food comes with wonderful memories. I remember on cold and wintry Sunday mornings my mother would make homemade chicken noodle soup. The windows would soon be wet with dew, and aroma would fill the house and always warm my heart and soul. I love chicken noodle soup. List your favorite food and why.

Favorite Things

"Frankly My Dear, I Don't Give a Damn."

When I need a good cry I watch *Steel Magnolias*. When I am in the mood for a musical I watch *Funny Girl*. When I want a good action movie I watch an "Indiana Jones" flick. List your favorite movies or theatre productions—ones that make you laugh, cry, put you on the edge of your seat or simply entertain you. Remember to add new ones.

Favorite Things

Friends Are Forever

Friendship implies loyalty, affection, sympathy, readiness to help, sticks with you, fights with and for you and never judges you. Make a list of people you call friend; someone who makes you laugh, someone who listens...someone who cares about you despite the fact they know everything about you!

There is nothing on this earth more to be prized than true friendship.

—St. Thomas Aquinas

Favorite Things

"You Ain't Nothin' but a Hound Dog"

Music can affect you in many different ways. When I hear "Mony, Mony," or "In the Mood" I gotta get up and dance! When I hear "I Got Friends in Low Places" or "Achy Breaky" I want to sing along...the trouble is I cannot carry a tune at all! When I hear "Amazing Grace," "In the Garden" and "How Great Thou Art," I feel blessed. I love music—all kinds of music.

List your all-time favorite songs and why. Add to the list as you hear new ones.

Favorite Things

Pets—Past, Present and in the Future

I will never forget one day when I was home alone feeling quite sorry for myself and crying my eyes out in the bathroom, I opened the door to find Katie our cat waiting at the door. She followed me into the bedroom and when I sat down on the bed she jumped up and proceeded to give me "cat kisses" as if to she was trying to console me.

List your favorite pets and what endeared you most to them. If you have never had a pet, list what animals you finding most interesting and why.

Favorite Things

"It Was the Best of Times; It Was the Worst of Times."

When I was younger one of favorite things to do was to grab a sack of seeds, a Mountain Dew, and a good book. I would literally sit for hours upon hours and read. Books are absolutely wonderful!

List your favorite books, the authors and why you liked them. List the books you would like to read someday. When you are finished reading it, add new ones to your list.

Favorite Things

"Did You Hear the One About..."

Have you ever heard a joke or story that made you laugh and then when you want to tell it to someone else you forget the punch line or the best part of the story? Write down your favorite jokes or stories. Remember...add new ones when you hear one!

Things I Want to Do Before I Die

Years ago I read an article in *Reader's Digest* called "Fifty Things I want to do before I die." It gave me the opportunity to think about some of the things I really want to do before I leave this earth.

Take a moment and think about what you would like to accomplish, try, taste, see, hear or feel before you are called home. As you make your list include why you think you can do it or why you think you cannot do it. You might discover there may be no obstacles in your way!

All About Me

Always Speak Well of Yourself

Did you know you think thousands and thousands of thoughts a day, and most of those thoughts are negative? "I can't do that; it's too hard." "I am never lucky." "I hate my job." "No one appreciates what I do," etc. It is referred to as self-talk. It is the conversation you carry on with you at all times.

And did you know that through your self-talk you trigger pictures in your mind, and those pictures or images bring about feelings and emotions?

Picture it this way.

Self-Talk
How I talk or affirm to myself
when I react to my own
evaluation or others'
evaluation of my performance

      REINFORCES

Self-Image
What I believe is true
about me and what I
think is good enough
for me.

      CONTROLS

It's just like me. I failed again.

I am so stupid.

I can't do anything right.

Why am I so dumb?

Performance Realty
How I act and perform based on
my current self-image.

STIMULATES

either positive or
negative **Self-Talk.**

Nobody likes me.

I hate my job.

I am afraid.

Self-Talk
How I talk or affirm to
myself
when I react to my own
evaluation or others'
evaluation of my
performance

I'll never learn how.

…and the cycle is
repeated.

To put it simply: *WHAT YOU THINK IS WHAT YOU GET!*

The Self-Talk Challenge: Become aware of your self-talk, negative and positive. Keep track of your self-talk by writing down your self-talk for one week. Discover what you are telling yourself. Change your negative self-talk into positive. You can do it! After all, you are a bright and capable person.

Praising Yourself

What you achieve is for you. Recognize and acknowledge your value. List things that you have achieved that have made you feel proud.

Let People Know How You Expect to Be Treated

Honoring is a decision to place high value, worth and importance on oneself and others. It is a decision to view oneself and others as a priceless gift.

List at least ten characteristics you honor about yourself.

1.
2.
3.
4.
5.
6.
7.
8.
9.
10.

Can you identify more? Super!

Whom do I want to recognize and honor daily?

What can I do differently to show someone that you honor him or her?

Always Picture in Your Mind How You Want It to Be— Not How It Really Is

What do you believe you can make happen for you? Do you have a clear vision of how you want it to be? Remember—Only you are responsible for your happiness and your life.

What do you want your life to look? As you write down what you want you life to look like be very explicit. Use colorful adjectives in you description. Be very precise. Reread what you have written over and over again. Also make changes when you need to…remember the only certainty in life is change.

Today I am feeling:

Today I am feeling:

Today I am feeling:

Today I am feeling: